D1507770

More than Movement for Fit to Frail Older Adults

Creative Activities for the Body, Mind, and Spirit

by

Pauline Postiloff Fisher, M.A.

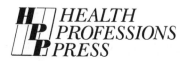

HEALTH PROFESSIONS PRESS

Baltimore • London • Toronto • Sydney

Health Professions Press, Inc.
Post Office Box 10624
Baltimore, Maryland 21285-0624

Copyright © 1995 by Health Professions Press.
All rights reserved.

Typeset by Signature Typesetting & Design, Baltimore, Maryland.
Manufactured in the United States of America by
The Maple Press Company, York, Pennsylvania.

First printing, February 1995
Second printing, April 1998

To purchase an audiotape to accompany this book or to inquire about workshop training, contact: Pauline Postiloff Fisher, A Moving Experience, 1884 Columbia Road, N.W., #105, Washington, DC 20009.

The videotape, *More Than Movement: Creative Activities for Older Adults*, is available from Health Professions Press. Call toll-free (888) 337-8808.

An earlier version of this book, *Creative Movement for Older Adults: Exercise for the Fit to Frail*, was published in 1989 by Human Sciences Press.

Note to readers: All exercise involves some risk. Before beginning any new physical activity, older people should consult their physicians.

Permission to reprint the following quotation is gratefully acknowledged: p. xix: Excerpted from *Maps to Ecstacy*, copyright 1989 by Gabrielle Roth. Reprinted with permission of Nataraj Publishing, 1561 S. Novato Boulevard, Novato, California 94947.

Library of Congress Cataloging-in-Publication Data

Fisher, Pauline P.
    More than movement for fit to frail older adults : Creative activities for the body, mind, and spirit / by Pauline Postiloff Fisher.
        p.   cm.
    Includes bibliographical references and index.
    ISBN 1-878812-21-1
    1. Exercise for the aged.   2. Physical fitness for the aged.   3. Aged–Recreation.   I. Title
GV482.6.F47   1995
613.7'0446—dc20   94-41602
                                                                                          CIP

British Library Cataloguing-in-Publication data are available from the British Library.

Contents

About the Author

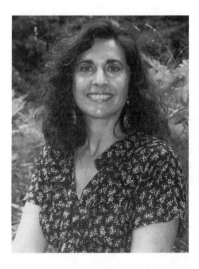

Like Shakespeare, I believe that "all the world's a stage" and that life is, as Baba Ram Dass (Richard Alpert) said, "the only dance there is." I find that if there's something you want to do, you may not do it; but if there's something you need to do, some how, some time, you will find the way to do it.

Dance was not something I wanted to do; it was something I had to do. Through dance one becomes more fully alive—physically, emotionally, intellectually, and spiritually. It opens a path toward one's higher self—a way to transcend the mundane.

As a result of my parents' discouragement, I wasn't able to begin formal dance training until age 12. By the age of 15, I began teaching dance at a community center to earn money to take more classes. My dance training has continued throughout my life and I came to realize later that life itself was, and continues to be, my greatest teacher.

It was as a dance education major that I entered Temple University in 1972. Then, because one of my sons had a learning disability—or learning difference, as I prefer to call it—I began to explore the use of dance with students with learning disabilities and other special children. This was my first exposure to the field of dance therapy. Later, I became aware that I also had learning differences, and there seems no doubt that dance training helped to improve my attention span, sequencing, visual perception, auditory perception, problem solving, and organization of thought.

The years in college opened my exploration into other areas of learning, such as meditation, yoga, psychology, theater improvisation, Tai Chi, creative visualization, body/mind theories, relaxation, and stress reduction techniques. I soon gave up teaching ballet, modern dance, and Slimnastics, but continued to teach creative movement education to children and adults, using dance and interrelated arts to teach curriculum and to enhance self-concepts, as well as working with special populations in therapeutic dance. I developed workshop programs called "A Moving Experience."

Some of these workshops explored the connection between body and mind, movement and emotions. They helped people to comprehend their personalities better through the ways in which they move, as well as to expand their movement vocabularies and improve awareness, awakening the child within through arts, play, and fun, while releasing joy.

In 1981 came an artist-in-residence grant from the Georgia Council for the Arts and Humanities. Although I had organized performance programs for older adults in Pennsylvania during the 1960s, it was during that time in Georgia that I first experienced teaching older adults and discovered what a delight it was. The residency required the creation of new dances. One of those pieces, created in memory of my grandmother, became the basis for "Particinformances." These were participatory, informal, informative performances that I did for nursing homes, veterans' hospitals, and other adult facilities around the country.

Other special constituent grants I received from the D.C. Commission on the Arts and Humanities were for intergenerational projects I designed for older adults and elementary children.

Besides my work with fit to frail older adults, I continue to work with others, including special populations. My staff trainings around the country include stress management and are presented in workshops, seminars, and courses for health care professionals and educators. I feel fortunate to be doing what I love and enriched by being able to share it.

Pauline Fisher

Foreword

More than Movement for Fit to Frail Older Adults: Creative Activities for the Body, Mind, and Spirit offers an abundance of original information that will be of tremendous help to activity directors, art therapists, therapeutic and recreation personnel—anyone serving both the fit and the frail. The book will be a boon to those who work at senior centers, adult day care programs, and long-term care facilities.

In seeking to accomplish her main goal—to get people moving—Pauline Fisher offers a wide range of activities to get a body in motion. With caution to do only what feels right and to pay attention to one's own abilities, Fisher suggests that, through movement, self-confidence can be gained, stress can be reduced, creative abilities can be awakened, and a connection can be made with our spiritual selves. Oh, yes—and it can all be fun as well!

Written with extraordinary sensitivity, her book is a unique resource for those working with both older adults and others. Pauline Fisher knows her stuff. Yet, she delivers far more than information on movement, exercise, and keeping the body fit. She teaches techniques that truly consider the whole person, not just specific body parts. With wit and wisdom, the chapters of the book unfold to reveal a message that nurtures the creative spirit and nourishes the soul.

Connie Goldman
Connie Goldman Productions, Inc.
Santa Monica, California

Preface

There are only two ways to live your life. One is as though nothing is a miracle. The other is as though everything is.

—Albert Einstein

*M*ore than Movement for Fit to Frail Older Adults describes a program I use with older adults and other groups of people with special needs. The main goal of the program is to get all people—from the very fit to the very frail—moving in whatever way they can while they have fun and learn that almost any movement can be dance. If you care about people and are sensitive to individual needs, the activities in this book will guide you, even if you have no prior experience or knowledge of working with older adults.

The program differs from some other movement and exercise programs in that it includes participants at every level and allows each participant to work at his or her own level of capability and comfort. The program stresses concern for the individual and the connections among the body, the mind, and the spirit. It engages not only the body but also the emotions and the intellect as well. I strongly believe in a higher source that guides our spiritual selves and find that the participants in my workshops respond to and appreciate the inclusion and recognition of that part of themselves.

The activities described in this book have been used at nursing homes, adult day care centers, senior centers, nutrition sites, hospitals, mental institutions, rehabilitation centers, retirement apartment complexes, Elderhostels, and other settings. They have been used with well older adults, people in wheelchairs, people in chronic pain, and people with severe cognitive impairment. I have also developed intergenerational programs, which include children of all ages. I vary my approach and focus depending upon the needs of each group.

The More than Movement program includes movement, dance, music, art, poetry, imagery, deep breathing and relaxation techniques, sensitivity awareness, theater games, communication motivators, and memory reinforcements, as well as laughter and readings or sharings to uplift the spirit. All the activities are enjoyable, creative processes that build participants' self-confidence while helping them become more aware of their bodies and themselves so that they feel better, both physically and mentally.

The specific goals of *More than Movement for Fit to Frail Older Adults* are to

- Motivate older adults to move
- Foster the ability to express oneself creatively
- Awaken sometimes dormant creative abilities
- Increase joint and body part articulation
- Improve body image and enjoyment of creative movement
- Enhance awareness through development of perceptual skills and reawakening of the senses
- Acquire techniques for relaxation and stress management
- Improve memory and communication skills
- Facilitate social interaction
- Use the arts and positive thought to uplift the whole person
- Have fun and laugh

To facilitate the program effectively, it is important to be as flexible and patient as possible, and to be aware that the conditions under which you work may often be less than optimal. My own teaching experiences have included holding classes in the following venues:

- A retirement apartment complex where the group met in an open space next to the lobby. (I tried to look at the positive side of this experience, which was that some of those passing through became interested and joined the group.)
- Wards of hospitals or nursing homes where the loudspeaker periodically interrupted our class.
- The activity room of an apartment complex that was often too hot or too cold.
- A recreation and nutrition center where there was only one large area, in which our class was held in the midst of other activities, including lunch setup.

Some facilities may be so understaffed that you may need to gather the residents yourself. Telephones may ring; visitors or other residents may walk in and out of the room in which you are teaching; a fire drill may interrupt your class; and the only chairs available may be soft chairs that you sink into. It is important to recognize that the goals of the program must be flexible and may need to be changed. Don't be disappointed if you don't get the response you had expected; try to be adaptable and patient and to retain a sense of humor.

The attitude of the group facilitator is critical to the success of the program. If the facilitator approaches the program as nothing more than a way to fill time and keep a group occupied, that attitude will be projected, and participants will get little pleasure from the program. Feel comfortable with your own body and select activities that you really enjoy doing. Try the activities before you present them to a group, find which activities you like best, and interact with participants with the enthusiasm and joy with which this program is meant to be presented. The appreciation I receive while sharing my own joy is a blessing.

Be honest with yourself and the group, believe in what you are doing, be able to do it yourself, and don't be afraid of trying something new. Before beginning a class, take a deep breath, tune into your heart, and remember to relax and have fun.

Acknowledgments

This book could not have been written without the knowledge and inspiration I received from all those who have touched my life and from whom I have learned.

I give thanks to all of my students, who helped me develop into the teacher I am today. I especially thank all my classes whose photos and stories help to make up this book.

To David Sparkman, my friend who helped me with the editing and advice on the original manuscript and the first draft of this edition, goes my deepest gratitude for his time, patience, moral support, sense of humor, and friendship.

To my friend Rebecca Vaughan, for her peaceful place in the mountains where I wrote the first draft of this edition and for her being who she is.

To Mark Shecter, for his friendship and support.

To my friend Ellen Maidman, who was on the other end of the phone, ready to listen and to make suggestions.

To my new friend, John Brackett, who took some of the photographs in this book.

And to all of my family and friends who encouraged and believed in me. I thank you.

This book is dedicated to

the memory of my father, Nathan Postiloff, who came to this country and persisted in making his dreams come true;

to my mother, Bertha Postiloff, who was his spirit, his love, and his partner in achieving those dreams;

and to my sons, Jeff, Russ T., and Kevin, who continually keep me in my heart and on my toes.

When I dance, I break free. I make up my own steps, let the beat all the way into my soul. I ride on the waves of music like a surfer. I bump against parts of myself, go between, around, stretch what I know. I go where I've never been. Through dance I've journeyed through my body into my heart, past my mind into another dimension of existence, a dimension I call ecstasy, total communion with the spirit.

—Gabrielle Roth, *Maps to Ecstasy*

More than Movement for Fit to Frail Older Adults

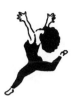

PART I
MOVEMENT ACTIVITIES

Chapter 1

Getting Started

Old age is ready to undertake tasks that youth skirted because they would take too long.

—Somerset Maugham

W orking creatively with older adults can be an exciting challenge, as well as a rewarding experience. Activities can help bring people out of themselves, making them feel good and improving their self-esteem.

To be effective with a group of older people, remember that:

- Many older people have hearing difficulties, so speak up, or seat a person with a hearing impairment next to you.
- Some older people have visual impairment, so you may need to demonstrate an activity at close range.
- Not all individuals will be dressed comfortably or properly for free movement and exercise. (The female residents of one retirement home arrived at every session in dresses, girdles, stockings, and heels, and would not have thought of dressing otherwise.)
- Very confused people may ramble on, or give incoherent or inappropriate responses. Some may try to put props in their mouths.
- Older people's energy level is lower in the afternoon. A few may fall asleep, either because they are on medication or because they are tired.
- It is a good idea to try to do each of the activities as you read them. Before presenting them to a group, experience the activities in your body and not just in your head. It may be

helpful to "rehearse" the activities with an aide, if you have one, or with a support group or network of other activity professionals.

• With the very frail or very confused, relax, go slowly, and have no expectations.

To begin, arrange the group and yourself in a circle of chairs. Move around among the group members. Go to those who need assistance with an activity, either directing or moving their bodies gently or placing their arms or other body parts correctly for them. For those who cannot move, give them the feeling of movement by moving a body part for them or holding their hands and moving with them very gently. Be sure that you establish one-on-one contact with each person in the group at least once during each session, and be sure to offer frequent praise. Reassure and compliment the participants without being patronizing.

Before beginning a new class, tell all participants to do only what feels right, to pay attention to their own body's abilities. Remind them that the purpose of the session is pleasure, not pain.

Try to create an atmosphere in which participants feel free to communicate with one another. When verbal interactions occur, it is easier to get people moving. The converse is also true—after movement activities, there is generally more verbal communication among the participants.

Sometimes older people are reluctant to participate in a group. One woman at a retirement home complained of dizziness and a headache and asked if she could watch the group rather than participate in it. After several minutes of sitting on the sidelines, she forgot her dizziness and headache and ended up participating fully. The color in her face changed, and so did her energy level. Just leaving her room, where she had been all alone, and joining others had proved beneficial.

Reluctance to join a group sometimes reflects the fear of recognizing the child within ourselves. Older people who will eagerly get down on the floor to play with their grandchildren may find it difficult to get down on the floor to play with the child within themselves. Regardless of our age, there are child-like qualities that we never want to lose—curiosity, imagination, playfulness, open-mindedness, willingness to experiment, eagerness to learn, awe, living in the present, forgiveness, the need to love, humor, energy, and honesty. We do not stop playing when we grow old—we grow old when we stop playing.

For many adults, reluctance to play reflects the fact that they have been serious all their lives and have not had the opportunity to play or to be self-expressive with the arts. Even in the corporate world, play and humor are used to jog people's thinking out of the predictable and already tried. Painting to music, dressing as clowns, and even having clients imagine themselves as telephones have all been used.

ENERGY AND MOTIVATION

When I teach, I am totally involved in what I am doing and the people I am with. I am in the moment. I am comfortable with myself, with what I am doing, and with the group. It is natural for me to remain continually relaxed yet active. Without being frantic or overexcited, I maintain a stimulated, attentive attitude. Giving of myself comes across, and I end up infecting others with my energy. Even when I sometimes feel tired or low before teaching, once I start to teach—giving and receiving—I am uplifted. No matter what is going on in my life, I enter a room for a group session with a positive attitude. Like an actress going on stage, once I begin a session I change roles. I am not acting, however—I *am* that person.

Remember, energy creates more energy—a good mood is transmitted. There are times, however, when things that are askew in my life are strongly on my mind. At such times, I simply share my feelings with the group so that we can look at the similarities in our humanness. This is stimulating to the group and promotes social interaction. I end up looking at my own problems from a distance. Sometimes we can laugh together at ourselves.

It is the responsibility of the group facilitator to keep the energy level of a group up, especially with older adults who are in pain or depressed. When I was teaching at a hospital geriatric unit, one man in a wheelchair was wheeled in. Angrily, he announced that he was in pain, and that he was not going to move. Once the group got started, however, and he was able to put aside his pain, he found himself becoming involved in the activities. Later, he indicated that he had enjoyed himself, something that was clearly visible. The enthusiasm of the facilitator and of the other group participants can make everyone feel better.

USING MUSICAL INSTRUMENTS TO BREAK THE ICE

One way of beginning a class is to pass around a musical instrument—a tambourine, cymbals, a drum. When instruments are not available, you can make your own. Beans can be put in a jar, an empty coffee can may be used as a tom-tom, keys can be jangled. If the instrument is an unusual one, talk about it first, explaining to the group that, even if they don't know how to play the instrument, they can play with it. Ask each person to do whatever he or she would like on the instrument and then say his or her name. This activity is fun and helps to bring the class together. It helps to bring us into the present, leaving behind where we've just been, or where we are going next, helping us to focus on the moment.

Most people don't get the opportunity to experience musical instruments personally—to handle instruments and to make music themselves. The experience of making music can be gratifying, and often provokes joyous smiles. For the very frail, it is a motivator for minimal movement. Saying our names is a way of saying, "Hi, this is me and I'm here." It also reminds us of and reinforces the names of everyone in the group. This is a reinforcement for the facilitator as well as for the members of the group. In too many facilities, participants do not know each other by name. Often it is because they forget, but sometimes it reflects the lack of intimacy among the residents.

Eye contact is very important for connection while talking to another person. When moving from person to person, kneel in front of each person so that you are on the same level as they are in their chairs. With people with cognitive impairment who do not respond to their names, take their hand and hit the instrument, saying their name for them while looking into their eyes.

RHYTHM SOUNDS AND GROUP ECHO

Another way to begin a session is for each person to choose a rhythm and have the group echo by clapping the rhythm back. This activity is also helpful as a listening exercise. The rhythm can be one of the individual's own design. If someone has difficulty, I suggest using the rhythm (by syllables) of one's full name or birth date. For example, *Mary Ann Peterson* has six beats; the rhythm would be as it is said: -- - ---. Several such rhythms can be put together into a song and then movement can be added.

MUSIC SELECTION

Music selection is an important part of a movement program. I try to start with music that each group can relate to, by using music that was popular when the group was younger and music that appeals to the particular ethnic group with which I may be working. From that point, I add a variety of music, introducing new musical selections to expand the musical knowledge of each group.

Throughout the book I make some suggestions about music, but I encourage all group facilitators to explore different kinds of music on their own. Check what you have at home or what is available in the facility in which you are working. Other good sources are the public library and the music libraries of your friends. A list of suggested music is provided at the end of the book in Appendix A.

DEEP BREATHING AND BREATH AWARENESS

After name introductions, a class can start with deep breathing. Deep breathing brings oxygen to the lungs and helps activate the diaphragm, which in turn helps take in more oxygen. In this way, the lungs get rid of carbon dioxide and other waste products. This process induces relaxation and helps you feel better. Deep breathing and breath awareness can be facilitated by blowing soap bubbles, blowing out the flame of a candle, blowing enough to make a pinwheel spin, and/or blowing a balloon off someone's hand. Each of these calls for a different kind of breath, such as slow and long, or short and fast.

Soap Bubbles

Soap bubbles are both pretty and fun. Quite often a member of the group who rarely participates in other activities will blow bubbles. This activity calls for a long, slow breath (Figure 1). For some very frail older people, this may be difficult. This activity can be extended by using music and having each person break the bubbles with a different body part. One person can blow the bubbles while another dances the bubbles away, breaking them with as many body parts as possible, using the legs and head as well as the elbows and feet. The music and bubbles motivate the other group members to cheer them on. For the very frail, the group facilitator can blow the bubbles. If they can respond, they can break the bubbles or they can blow them back. If they do not respond, the facilitator might blow the bubbles on their hands or arms so that they can feel the sensation of them breaking. This can be done for people with severe visual impairment as well.

In another variation, each participant holds the bubble applicator in one hand, makes large arm movements that will blow the bubbles around, and then changes hands and repeats.

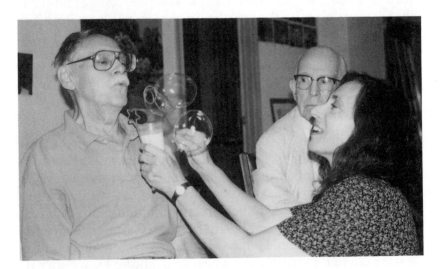

Figure 1.   Deep breathing can be stimulated by blowing soap bubbles.

Participants use both sides of their bodies if they can. If they cannot, they do the activity twice on one side. Music, such as a waltz, can motivate more dancelike movement.

This activity stimulates body part articulation and movement that is fun and more like dance than exercise. Although the attention is on breaking the bubbles, each person is moving and loosening muscles that may be stiff in his or her own way and at his or her own speed.

Candle Flame

Bring a candle in a holder to class. Light the candle for each person, asking each to make a wish before blowing out the candle (Figure 2). This takes a short and hard breath; some very frail group members may need assistance. If you are not permitted to use a flame, use a flashlight, which you can turn on and off when someone blows on it. Alternatively, hold a lit candle and have the whole group blow with you as you blow it out.

This activity could be extended into a memory recaller by asking if anyone remembers the first birthday candles he or she blew out, or any other happy memories associated with candles. Not only will this motivate sharing and communication, but it may aid memory function as well.

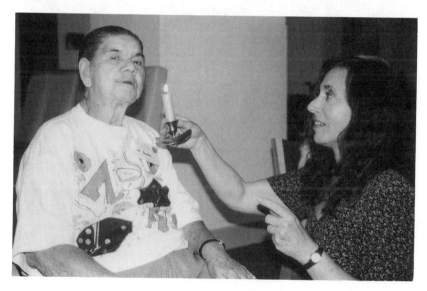

Figure 2.   Blowing out a candle requires a short, hard breath.

Pinwheels

Pinwheels can be introduced to generate a long and strong breath (Figure 3). Pinwheels are pretty and colorful and attract attention when they spin. Often the group may have to be reminded that they must blow into one of the pockets to get the pinwheel to spin; you may need to point out the pocket. Another activity using the pinwheel is to have each person stand, when possible, and dance as he or she moves the pinwheel through space with each arm in turn used to make it spin.

Balloons

Have each participant blow a balloon off your hand as you hold it near his or her mouth. If each person tilts his or her head toward the ceiling and you hold the balloon very gently between your hands close to the person's mouth, the balloon can be blown up toward the ceiling. (For variations of balloon activities see Chapter 5.)

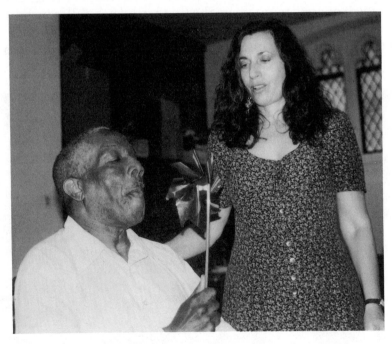

Figure 3. Blowing on a pinwheel can generate a long, strong breath.

Chapter 2

Making Music and Movement

There is nothing more remarkable in the life of Socrates than that he found time in his old age to learn to dance and play on instruments and thought it time well spent.

—Montaigne

Music and rhythm have been found to be very effective in reaching older adults with Alzheimer's disease. Music can have healing powers for most of us, but the results for those with dementia have been truly amazing. Neurologist Oliver Sacks believes that the right kind of music may even move those who can't walk to dance, those who can't speak to sing, and those who can't remember to remember.

People become more animated and alive through music and dance. I have witnessed nursing home residents who do not speak sing entire songs that they knew from their past. During a workshop with residents who used wheelchairs, one got up and danced in place with me as I held her hands. This woman had not stood in 3 years because of arthritis.

To be effective, music must be familiar. Music can bring memories of the times when the tunes were popular, and of the person's relationship to the music and the times. Music and dance are not cure-alls but, when used in conjunction with other modalities, can be very effective. Music inspires one to move, to participate, to come to life.

MUSIC AND MOVEMENT ACTIVITIES

Sing Alongs with Movement

Using songs such as "When Irish Eyes Are Smiling," "The Sidewalks of New York," "Bye, Bye Blackbird," "The Old Gray Mare," and "Little Brown Jug," clap out the rhythms and add different body movements with each line. You can use any song you'd like that would be familiar to the group. For example, the following body movements could be used with the song, "Bicycle Built for Two":

Song Line	Body Movement
1: *Daisy, Daisy, give me your answer do*	Sway upper body from side to side as arms sway in front of you from side to side.
2: *I'm half crazy, all for the love of you.*	Both hands touch heart, then reach up on right side; repeat touching heart and reach to left side.
3: *It won't be a stylish marriage,*	(Either sitting or standing) Step with the left foot and kick with the right foot, crossing over in front of the body to the left side; then step with the right foot and kick with the left foot, crossing over in front of the body to the right side.
4: *I can't afford a carriage.*	Clap, pat knees, clap.
5: *But you'll look sweet upon the seat*	Clap and reach right arm crossing in front of the body toward the left; clap and reach left arm crossing in front of the body toward the right.
6: *Of a bicycle built for two.*	Both arms open and reach out in front of the body, both touch the heart quickly, then open arms and reach out in front of the body again.

With repetitions of sentences or a phrase, repeat the same body movement. For participants with cognitive impairments, just hearing the song could be enough to get them to smile, or perhaps sway or stamp out the rhythm with their feet and just possibly to sing along.

Music and Movement

One way to combine music and movement is to break music into easily understood components. For example, composer Carl Orff devised a teaching method for children that uses body sounds such as hand clapping, knee slapping, finger snapping, or foot stomping as instruments. An example would be three quick hand claps, one slow knee slap with both hands, one finger snap with both hands.

Ostinato

One of the musical definitions used by Orff that you can use in class is ostinato, a rhythm or melody repeated continuously in the background while a speech or song is being performed. For example, one group can repeat "Bah, bah, bah, bah" slowly while another group recites or sings "Mary had a little lamb." Movement can be added by using the body as a musical instrument: Have one group continuously stomp their feet slowly if sitting, or one foot at a time if standing while a second group, in a faster rhythm, snaps their fingers once, slaps their knees once, and claps their hands twice, making the sounds "snap, slap, clap, clap."

Rondo

Rondo is one of the oldest musical forms. It involves repeating a rhythmic form in the pattern of A-B-A-C-A-D-A. A is always the same rhythm or movement, while B, C, and D are all different. An example of a rondo form would be: One person or one group claps out a waltz rhythm. This would be called A. B would be represented by another person or group stepping out a cha-cha rhythm. Then group A would clap out the waltz rhythm again. Then group C would stamp out a marching rhythm, and so on, as far as you would like to take it. A waltz rhythm is "slow, quick, quick," the same as clapping out the rhythm of the months Sep/tem/ber, Oc/to/ber, No/vem/ber, De/cem/ber. A cha-cha rhythm is = "slow, slow, quick, quick,

quick." This activity would be too complicated for persons with cognitive impairment, but perhaps they could participate in the ostinato rhythm.

Using these techniques, divide the group into smaller groups (or this can be done with the individuals), giving each a specific rhythmic pattern that either you or they have created. Using either real instruments or body instruments, set up an ostinato rhythm, such as a steady four-count beat. Then create either a song form or a rondo form.

Music, Math, and Movement

Give each person three pieces of construction paper. One piece represents a whole note (four counts). Suggest that they can divide the pieces any way they want—there is no set formula. Explain that a half piece of paper represents a half note, which equals two counts. Dividing the paper into four pieces would create four quarter notes of one count each. Each person can create a musical phrase using the construction paper and then add body movement. Some examples of the construction paper rhythms and body movements are:

Paper	Paper configuration representing musical phrase	Body movement corresponding to musical phrase
1		Lift right knee up on first count as you clap and lower on hold; repeat with left knee on second count as you clap.
2		Lift both arms up to ceiling on count of one as you clap and lower to the three remaining beats.

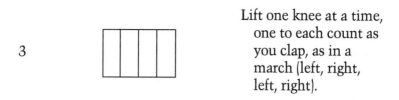

3   Lift one knee at a time, one to each count as you clap, as in a march (left, right, left, right).

These can be combined to form dances. The body movements can be performed in a sitting or standing position. Those participants who are not dancing with their whole bodies or body parts can play the rhythms on instruments or body instruments. This exercise would not be appropriate for persons with dementia.

Matching Movement with Rhythm

With participants who have a cognitive impairment, it is a good idea to match their movement and pace with a musical rhythm, accepting and allowing their timing. This can be done by clapping the rhythm, by using an instrument, or by finding appropriate music that you can play. Alternatively, you may start by mirroring one of their movements, such as a stomping foot or the action of a hand that is pulling on an article of clothing (without actually pulling), thus entering their world. After establishing their movement pattern and doing it for a few moments, you might then try to vary the movement slightly. An example would be adding a kick to a stamping foot (e.g., three stamps and one kick, and repeat) or adding the use of body instruments. These include such things as hand clapping, knee slapping, finger snapping, and foot stomping. These can be combined with the basic elements of musical rhythm and form. You might give the group a rhythm and ask them to use body instruments to perform. Or, you might ask them to make up a rhythm and body movement using body instruments. An example of this would be three quick hand claps, one slow knee slap with both hands, and one finger snap with both hands.

Chapter 3

The Elements
of Movement

I hear and I forget;
I see and I remember;
I do and I understand.

—Chinese proverb

The elements of movement are part of the vocabulary of dance. Just as baking and cooking have ingredients that make up each of the recipes, movement components are the ingredients that make up dances. Shape, space, time, and force are used by dancers, artists, and musicians alike. In dance and movement, we also use locomotor and nonlocomotor movement, and what I call energies.

This book is about being creative. It is important for every person who facilitates a group to decide whether the activities are appropriate for their group. That means that the activities described in this book are a jumping off point for each of you to change each activity to fit your specific needs. Because each group is as individual as each person, it is best for the facilitators to choose and perhaps vary the activities for their particular group. Often a group is mixed in abilities, both physically and mentally, so it is up to each facilitator to decide what to use and how. Before and during each session, remind participants to pay attention to their own bodies, to what feels comfortable and right for them.

SHAPE

Shape is the position the body or any body part takes in space. Shape can be explored in the following ways:

1. Make a shape with a specific body part, such as an arm or leg.
2. Make a shape with the whole body. First, assume a frozen pose, then find a way to move in this pose, either in place or through space (around the room).
3. Have a leader call out two or three body parts with which each participant can make a statue (frozen pose) or move in space.
4. Make a set of cards with names and possibly photographs from magazines, of various body parts. Have someone in the group pick a card, which will determine the body part that he or she will then touch to another body part. For instance, if a card with the word or picture of a nose is selected, the participant would walk around the room and touch the walls with his or her nose, or touch other people's noses. Or they may partner up and touch each other's noses. This game can be varied in many ways. If two cards are picked, participants may try to touch one body part to the other (e.g., touching a nose to a knee).

    For people with dementia in adult day care centers or long-term care facilities, pictures from magazines or any other photographs you may have may be used. Pick out the body parts, and then point to the same body parts on their bodies or while looking in a mirror. Be creative and make up your own games.
5. Make a shape with a body part and trace it on a piece of paper. Find a way of making shadows and make shadow shapes with body parts or the whole body.
6. Let participants form pairs. When given the signal, one partner makes a shape with the whole body. At a second signal, the other partner makes a shape while the first partner relaxes.

SPACE

Space is the area in which movement takes place. Space includes:

- *Path of movement* (e.g., straight [direct], or curved, twisted, crooked [indirect, flexible])—the road of travel, as Dorothy traveled the yellow brick road in *The Wizard of Oz.*
- *Direction*—the way the body is moving (e.g., forward; backward; sideways; diagonally; turning in, out, up, down).
- *Level*—the position of the body (e.g., prone, sitting, squatting, kneeling, standing, elevated). It also can be low, middle, or high.
- *Size of movement* (e.g., large, tall, wide, small, short, low, narrow).
- *Focus*—where the eyes look—constant in a particular direction, wandering, near, far, outward, or inward.

I suggest that you make a stack of cards for each of these elements of space so that you may mix these ingredients and make your own "recipes" (i.e., mix the elements to design your own activities). Here are a few of my ideas:

1. Choose some element of space for each body part to explore. For example, move elbows in the directions of front and back. Then do a large and high movement with an arm, exploring size. Follow this with a movement on a low level in a straight path while keeping the focus wandering, as if watching a butterfly fluttering around while crawling on your hands and knees.

2. Split the group in half so that partners are facing each other. Choose two directions, such as back and front, and a path, such as straight. Have half the group use their legs and the other half use their arms, and ask them to explore dancing in these directions and this path with the chosen body parts; then have the groups change body parts.

3. Call out a path and, at a signal, have participants change levels while continuing along the same path. At another signal, have them change the path while maintaining the same level. For instance, ask the group to walk a straight path and, at the beat of a drum or the clap of your hands, walk on tiptoes, or with knees bent. Or tell the group to walk a straight path while moving a body part in a curved pattern. For people who cannot walk, a straight path can be explored with an arm on a low level and then a high level.

4. Hold an object and move the object so that participants' eyes follow it. (I remember doing this at a nursing facility

with a resident with cognitive impairment. I was holding an object, trying to get her to move her head and look at the object high and low and side to side. No matter what I did, she did not respond. Finally giving up, I said, "Don't you want to move your head?" She responded by shaking her head from side to side, gesturing "No."] Sometimes, as facilitators, we try too hard. You may want to make a script: 1) "Look at the table, 2) the painting on the back wall, 3) the floor near your foot, 4) out the windows." Tell the group to walk with their focus wandering, with their focus far away, with their focus inward, and then straight ahead. This is great for sequencing and for listening to follow directions.

TIME

Time can be changed by changing the rate of speed (tempo) of movement—from slow to fast. Many activities can be explored or varied by changing the element of time. Music can be used to initiate this change. Dances can be set to a specific number of beats and then varied by changing the intervals between the beats. The following are some examples of how you can get the group to do this:

1. Have the group walk around the room three times, first very slowly, then a bit faster, and then as fast as they can.
2. Ask participants to move their arms in a circular path (pattern) very quickly. At a signal, have them move their arms in slow motion.
3. Have the group walk while keeping time with a slow count of four, or four slow claps. After four sets of four, change to four sets of a cha-cha rhythm (slow, slow, quick, quick, quick).

FORCE

Force (dynamics) describes the quality of movement—tense, heavy, hard, relaxed, soft, light, or weak. In order for the group to explore each of these forces, ask them to walk around the room, starting with a normal walk. Tell them that, at a given signal, everyone will stop. Then call out, "Walk tensed." At a predetermined signal, everyone will stop, and you can then call out, "Walk heavily." This process can continue until all of the elements of force have been explored. You may decide to explore just two each time you do this activity.

Another way to explore force would be to do a movement with a specific body part. Then choose a specific force, and repeat the movement with that force. For instance, you could ask the group to swing their arms front and back naturally, and then swing them heavily, as if each weighed a ton. Dramatic phrases are enhanced by the specific choices of the above elements.

ENERGIES

Energies is a term I use to describe movements that correspond to the musical terms *legato, staccato, vibratory, swinging,* and *percussive.* After explaining each of these terms, giving examples in visual images, sounds, and music, I ask the group to explore each with individual body parts. I then ask them to move the whole body in this energy. I also ask participants to pick a partner and have a short conversation speaking in a voice that corresponds to the type of energy that is being explored.

Types of Energies

Legato

Legato is constant, even-flowing movement. The sound of a constant hum is legato. It is usually done very slowly because it is more difficult to control when done quickly. There are no jerky movements in legato; movements are usually rounded and curved. Examples of visual images of legato are flowing water, the movement of wheat in a field, and astronauts in outer space.

Staccato

Staccato is short, fast, jerky movement, such as touching a hot iron or clapping your hands. Staccato movement is usually angular and sharp. It can be even or uneven in rhythm. Scattered dots on a piece of paper is a visual example of staccato.

Most disco music is staccato, and the sound of a train rolling across tracks or a ticking clock are examples of staccato sound. Authoritarian voices (e.g., military orders) and reprimanding voices (e.g., "Don't you ever do that again!") would be staccato voices.

Vibratory

There is a fine line between staccato and vibratory sound. Vibratory sound is much quicker than staccato sound. Shivering and rapid shaking, such as when someone is very cold or very nervous, are examples of vibratory movement. The movement can be tense or loose, such as the tight, quick movement of chattering teeth or the loose movement of an uncontrollable shake of Parkinson's disease. A jackhammer is a good example of a vibratory sound.

Swinging

Swinging is just that, movement that feels like being on a swing or pendulum. Swinging is giving in to gravity and suspending briefly in the air before falling back again. This is best explored by having everyone lift an arm in the air and let that arm fall in a swinging arc until it comes to a stop and suspends, before letting it fall and return again in an arc. This can be done with a feeling of falling and giving in to gravity, or with force, as if throwing the arm away or pitching a baseball underhand. Continual swinging movement often becomes circular. Scalloped edges and spirals are visual images of swinging. Waltz music is swinging. The stereotypical voice of a Southern belle or a whining child would be examples of voices that dip up and down in a swinging rhythm.

Percussive

Percussive sound is explosive, like a firecracker going off. Visually, it is like being shot out of a cannon, or a karate chop, quick and strong, strong enough to go through a wall. Much of the music of Bela Bartok and Darius Milhaud, for example, is percussive. Vocally imitating the sound of a gun shot is percussive.

Exploring Different Energies

Have the group explore each energy one at a time, first all together with the help of the facilitator making suggestions, and then each working alone during his or her own movement to that energy. Ask the group to add sounds that come out of the movement. You will find that each person's sound is as individual as his or her movement. Sometimes making sounds can be intimidating. You may want to find a way to gently encourage the people who might feel silly or uncomfortable, or tell them that making the sound is not compulsory.

At some point, when you feel it is appropriate (perhaps after 30–60 seconds or more), ask the group to freeze. Then choose a few people, one at a time, to make their sound. Let that be the "music" to which the rest of the group moves. After each sound, ask the group how this sound influenced their movement, and how it was different from their own movement and sound, even though it was the same energy. After the group has experienced the movements and sound of three to six people, ask which sounds felt comfortable, easy, or difficult for them. Ask them which sounds expanded their movement vocabulary.

Next, have everyone in the group choose a partner and explore a conversation using voices in a specific energy. If it is in legato, for example, each word will be slow, even, and somewhat drawn out, without inflection or any rise or fall in volume and with no tempo changes. After a minute or so, initiate a short discussion about feelings and perceptions. Ask how their individual conversations went and how the energy affected what they said and what was heard.

Another related activity is to have each person do a short everyday movement in mime, such as combing hair, brushing teeth, or eating, in the same natural energy that is normally used to perform such activities. Then ask each person to practice doing the same movement in two other energies, such as swinging and percussive. Let each person perform or demonstrate his or her movement before the group in three ways: first in the normal everyday energy and then in two other energies.

Ask each person to see how many energies he or she can do at the same time. In all my years of teaching I have seen only two people who could do all five at once, and both used batting of the eyelashes for the staccato movement. It takes some coordination even to use two or three together. It's like rubbing your stomach and patting your head at the same time. However, it is fun to try.

One more idea is to have everyone in the group pick a partner and stage a mock fight. The partners stand or sit far enough away from each other (without touching) so that they do not accidentally hurt each other. First, one partner socks, hits, punches, or kicks at the other without touching, like mirror or shadowboxing. Then the other partner responds in movement and with sound as if he or she were hit. Then the partner who responded reacts by punching or hitting back. The two partners continue to take turns as in a conversation or a real fight. This process can be done in one of the energies, or the facilitator can have the group freeze and then change from one energy to another. This activity works very well in legato, percussive, or staccato energies.

MOVEMENT ACTIVITIES

Nonlocomotor Movements

Nonlocomotor movements are movements that can be done in place or moving: bend, stretch, twist, swing, push, pull, dodge, strike, rock and sway, lift, sit, fall, bounce, and shake. Explore these movements one at a time, first with body parts and then with whole body movements. Musical instruments can accompany the activity, or appropriate music for each nonlocomotor movement may be used. I have also done this activity successfully with no music at all.

Body Part Articulation

Starting with bending, ask everyone to explore how many ways he or she can bend each body part, one body part at a time (e.g., bend the head to the front, back, and side; bend the fingers; bend the elbows; bend the torso to the front, back, and side). The facilitator may suggest ways to explore various movements or ask for suggestions. The group may also make its own choices of movements for exploration.

Statues

After body part articulation, ask each person to make a bent body statue using his or her whole body. At the sound of a drum or tambourine or a word signal, have each change the statue, and body level when applicable, at each beat.

Next, have one person go to the center of the room and make a bent body statue. One by one other group members then connect to one or more of the group in some way, until as many as 8–12 people are forming a group statue. Remind the group that the statue may be more interesting to look at if there are a variety of levels, with some people sitting, some standing, some kneeling, and some even lying down, as well as facing various directions (Figure 4). Encourage the group to make any shape other than a straight line.

For people who cannot stand or have difficulty standing, have them use their chairs or have the seated person be the first to start the statue. This process can be repeated for each nonlocomotor movement. A group statue can even combine a few different movements. For example, two people may bend, three stretch, and two twist.

I have done statues with people who are in wheelchairs. When it is a mixed group with one or two who are in wheelchairs, I move the people in wheelchairs to the center first and let them establish the beginning of the statue. The rest of the group then builds the statue from that point. When all of the

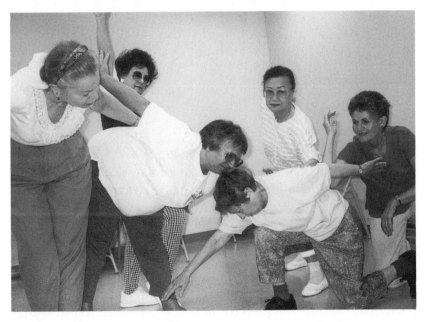

Figure 4.   Participants have a chance to bend and stretch while forming a group statue.

participants use wheelchairs, statues are more difficult to form, so we work in smaller groups of two or three.

Scripts

Each member of the group can choose three or four nonlocomotor movements and do each one in succession, like a script. Or, each person can pick three or four cards from a stack of cards, each one indicating the name of a nonlocomotor movement. This can be varied by, for example, doing all of the movements in legato, letting each statue pose flow into the next. Another variation is to change each pose at the beat of a drum or another signal. Transitions can be added in between each pose. For example, the participants could pose in a bend, then turn the whole body and pose in a stretch, then walk to another place and do a twist pose.

Nonlocomotor Movements Combined with Walking

Take four nonlocomotor movement cards and place each one in the center of the group, facing each of the four walls so that the cards form a small square. Have the group walk or dance around the room in any way they individually wish to. Use music with no particular beat that can serve to motivate but that will not necessarily influence each person's rhythm or speed, such as Kitaro's "Silk Road." The object is to touch each of the four walls with a different body part. After touching each wall, each person must come to the center next to one of the cards and do the corresponding nonlocomotor movement, holding it for three counts before going to the next wall. It is important that everyone moves at his or her own pace.

When participants have touched all four walls and done all four of the nonlocomotor movements, they can sit down. This is not a contest or race, just the fun of the process. In fact, you may add another element by having participants say hello as they pass each other, or freeze in their last pose until all have finished. Or, at the beat of a drum, they may touch the person closest to them. If the group numbers 20 or more, you can break the group in half, so that each group can have a turn to participate and to watch. This activity is interesting to watch because it becomes a dance.

Locomotor Movements

Locomotor movements include walking, running, jumping, and hopping. Other locomotor movements tend to be combinations or variations of these movements. For example, leaping is a variation of running, and a skip is a combination of a step and a hop.

A fun way to get a group moving is to create a deck of cards, each indicating a different locomotor movement. Ask each participant to throw a die and pick a card from the stack. The locomotor movement indicated on the card is then performed the number of times that comes up on the die. A variation is to pick three or four cards and throw the die for each one. This becomes a script of a short phrase or the beginning of a dance, which can then be performed to one piece of music, such as a waltz. This same script will totally change if done to another piece of music, such as disco or a march.

Another variation is to have one stack of cards, each containing a nonlocomotor movement, and another stack of cards, each containing an emotion. A third stack of cards can contain descriptive action words. Each person picks a card from each stack and simultaneously demonstrates the movement, emotion, and action that are indicated on the cards. An example of the three cards picked might be *twist, angrily,* and *fast.* Be aware that the word perform might intimidate some. Demonstrating alone might be fearful for some people, in which case you can suggest that two or three people work together, or have the whole group do it at one time. Sometimes, members of the group will come up with more ways to vary an activity creatively.

Laban Effort/Shape

A useful tool for creating and exploring movement is Laban Effort/Shape, which was developed by Rudolf von Laban (1879–1958). This system is used to observe, analyze, and define all elements of human movement, and it is applied to art, education, recreation, dance therapy, and industry. Laban Movement Analysis examines the interrelatedness of the body, the effort flow of movement, and the use of space.

The vocabulary terms of the system include *effort flow* (flow) and *effort qualities* (space, force or weight, and time).

Many dancers use this vocabulary as a method for choreography.

Effort flow changes tension, or energy in the body, from free to bound. Free flow movement is light and, at its extreme, would be so light it would float away. It is movement without stress, whereas bound movement is tight and, at its extreme, would condense so tightly into itself it would also disappear, like a black hole.

Have the group experiment with flow using different body parts, starting with the arms. Suggest that they start with free flow movement, using the image of a feather floating in the air. Tell them to slowly place more and more tension into their arms and the movement until the arms and movement become so tight that they contract into a ball close to the body. Bound movement can be explained as a tautness or even rigidity in movement. For example, tell the members of the group to allow an arm to relax and slowly and gently begin to close the fingers and then the hand until they make a fist as tight as possible. Picking up something even as light as a feather or piece of paper requires a certain amount of muscle tension.

Space is either direct, which is single, focused, and a straight line, or indirect, which is meandering, twisting, avoiding, unable to hold at any point—it may be several parts of the body going in different places at the same time.

To explore a *direct* path in space, suggest that the class experiment walking a direct line from one point in the room to another, deciding ahead of time where the two points will be. The facilitator can determine the starting and ending point or each person in the class can make that decision for himself or herself. For those who are unable to stand or move around, the direct line can be made with an arm, a leg, or even the head.

To explain an *indirect* path in space, throw a feather in the air, have two or more people blow on it as it makes its descent, and watch the indirect path it makes on its journey down. The images of a bee or fly buzzing around or a butterfly flitting about are also good examples. Almost everyone has seen a comedian depicting an inebriated person stumbling around, unable to walk a direct path. Ask for volunteers to demonstrate an indirect path in space either with a body part or by moving the whole body through space.

Force is a change in effort from *light,* which is buoyant and yielding, to *strong,* which is firm movement with a forceful intention. A ball floating buoyantly in a calm, undulating sea of water is a good example. Ask the group for other images that would be examples of light, and then have everyone explore light movement with one or more body parts. For strong movement, describe or demonstrate a karate kick. Or, give each person the opportunity to put his or her fist through a piece of paper (Figure 5) large enough for two people to hold firmly and straight, but not too tautly, one person on each side of the participant, so that he or she can strike through the paper in a strong way using force.

Time ranges from sustained movement, like that of a lava light or an arm that moves slowly upward like an unfolding flower, to sudden movement, like an explosion or an arm that is held up and then drops quickly down.

Combinations of these basic efforts would be:

Float—light + slow + indirect, like a feather or balloon floating in a breezy wind. An example of a floating movement could be arms that move from one side to another like the undulating waves.

Dab—light + quick + direct, like tapping powder on with a powder puff. Have the class experiment in dabbing movements with different parts of their bodies, such as the head making movements like a woodpecker pecking at a tree.

Glide—light + slow + direct, like a blimp moving through the sky. In a sitting position, have everyone use slow skating motions with their legs.

Flick—light + quick + indirect, like the flutter of a bird's wings. Ask the class to pretend they are watching the path of a butterfly in the air and allow their heads to move quickly as their eyes dart up, right, up, left, down, up, etc., following the quick movements of the butterfly. Then ask them to explore this kind of movement with other parts of their bodies.

Punch—strong + quick + direct, like stomping on a bug. Punching can be explored with parts of the body other than the arm. Have participants, carefully, try punching with a leg, a hip, or the head.

Slash—strong + quick + indirect, like shooing a fly off your face. Suggest the participants pretend they are moving through a cave with many cobwebs. They can slash with their arms or elbows to move the cobwebs aside.

Press—strong + slow + direct, like pushing against a heavy revolving door. Have participants try this with different body parts. They may even try doing this with partners; explain that the object is not to press the partner off balance, but just to feel the pressure of each other's pressing.

Wring—strong + slow + indirect, like twisting the water out of a bathing suit. Tell the members of the group to hold one arm out in the air and slowly twist it in one direction and then the other, feeling a sense of a wringing motion.

Shape The shape qualities are similar to those suggested in the open/close activity in Chapter 6 and can also be explored in the same way as nonlocomotor movements.

Shape flow includes growing and shrinking. Shape qualities are horizontal, vertical, and sagittal. *Horizontal* goes from

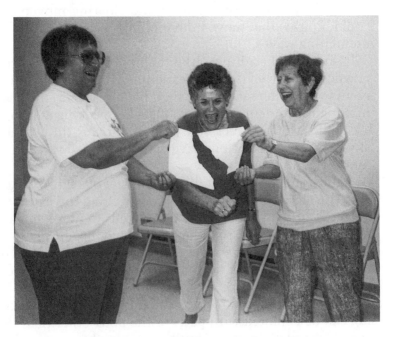

Figure 5. A demonstration of force.

widening (sideward out) to narrowing (sideward across). Have the class members experience these by stepping out and reaching out, feeling the sense of the side-to-side horizontal space. Follow this by asking them to cross one foot over the other and one arm over the other and feel the narrowness of their bodies in space. Have a discussion about things or people that move in these ways, or reasons for having to move in these ways.

Vertical goes from rising (upward) to shrinking (downward). Talk about things in nature that move in these ways, and then ask for some participants to demonstrate a few in pantomime, such as a tree growing straight up or a snowman melting.

Sagittal goes from advancing (forward) to retreating (backward). Divide the class in half and have them walk toward each other from opposite sides of the room and then, if appropriate, walk carefully backward. Or, the facilitator can move toward each person in the group and then move away, and ask each to describe his or her changing perceptions and feelings. This can lead into further discussions about memories involving people or things that have moved closer or further away, like a loved one leaving on a train.

Chapter 4

Ideas for Dances

*The living have danced from the beginning of time. I might
even say, the dance and life have moved along together.*
                                                    —Unknown

After the class has come together in whatever method
you have chosen (e.g., passing a musical instrument
around, clapping names), done some deep breathing, and completed a general body part warm-up, the group can begin to participate in some of the creative exercises presented here. These
activities can be repeated as appropriate, extended, and developed over time.

NAME WITH MOVEMENT

A good way to start with a new group is with an activity that
uses movement that gives all participants the opportunity to
present themselves by saying their names. First, ask each member of the group to state his or her first name. Participants who
are physically able to do so should then perform a movement
with an individual body part or with their whole body. To
familiarize the group with the names of all of its members, the
entire group repeats each member's name twice, performing
each person's body movement as the name is repeated. Group
members who are not able to imitate a particular movement
can simply repeat the person's name. This activity helps reinforce names for both the facilitator and the group members,
and it gives each person a chance to see how his or her own

movement looks on other people, as well as to see variations of the movement.

It is essential that the facilitator accept all movement variations and establish an environment that says, "You're okay, whatever you do is acceptable, you can be creative." People take risks by representing themselves with a movement. They may feel vulnerable expressing their creativity in front of a group. It is the responsibility of the facilitator to make certain that all group members feel successful within the group. By creating a nonthreatening atmosphere, the facilitator makes the class a safe place to be—a place in which people can be themselves, be silly, experiment creatively, and express themselves.

Depending on the number of people in each group and their capacity for remembering, the body movements used in this exercise can be strung together into a dance by adding music. Further refinement of the dance can be achieved by adding variations of each movement and transitions between movements, and by placing people in various formations as they perform.

GUIDED BODY PART DANCES

When members of the group are unable to propose movements themselves, the facilitator can guide the group by asking each person in the group to make a movement with a particular body part. For example, the facilitator can ask the first person in the circle to make a head movement, the next person a neck movement, the next person a shoulder movement, and so forth. Each time a new movement is added, the entire series of movements is repeated, encouraging both physical and mental effort. Any movement can be interpreted as appropriate. For example, if a participant shrugs his or her shoulders, this can be taken as a movement. If someone is stuck and cannot come up with a movement, the facilitator can suggest a movement.

When every group member has been included, all of the movements can be put together with fast upbeat music and "danced." Music with a distinct beat, such as disco music, is recommended. The dance can then be repeated in a different tempo to music with a different beat, such as blues.

CATEGORY DANCES

Dances can be developed around any category or topic, including sports, birthdays, picnics, or trips to the beach. For example, the facilitator might suggest that the group think about spending a day on the beach. Group participants can suggest the kinds of activities that are done at the beach (e.g., putting on suntan lotion, swimming, playing volleyball, looking for seashells). The facilitator should ask the group to perform the movements associated with each beach activity. As each new movement is added, the entire sequence of movements should be repeated and music should be added. For participants who are unable to stand, the resulting dance can be done in a seated position using as many body parts as possible.

Categories that are particularly appropriate for active groups are sports (Figure 6), housework, and farming. Two or three sports can be combined by using movements from each (e.g., pitching, batting, and running from baseball; kicking, throwing, and catching from football). Men particularly enjoy sports-related movements.

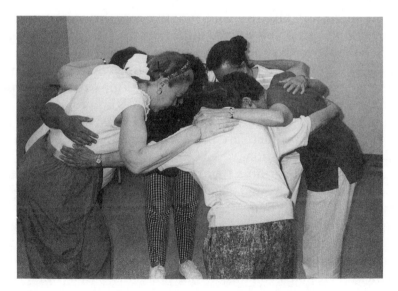

Figure 6. A category dance develops around a football huddle.

MOVEMENT AND EMOTIONS

Many older adults often do not have the opportunity to discuss emotions, particularly feelings that may be related to aging. Sharing these feelings in a safe environment, with a group of their peers, is a liberating experience. Being able to "dance" these emotions can release tension related to specific emotions that may be locked up.

Suppressed emotions may eventually affect body movement. Tightening of the body, for example, may be a result of blocking expressions of feeling. Chronic muscle tension can affect breathing and result in binding energy. Wilhelm Reich (1957) referred to this muscular tension as *armoring*. Wherever this chronic tension is held in the body, it looks and feels like an armored plate. In his book, *Bioenergetics*, Alexander Lowen describes how these muscle tensions begin:

> One inhibits the impulse to cry by setting the jaw, constricting the throat, holding the breath and tightening the belly. Anger as expressed in striking out can be inhibited by contracting the muscles of the shoulder girdle, thereby pulling the shoulders back. (1976, p. 144)

Expressing, sharing, and moving together can ease the sense of isolation and related emotions that older adults may feel. Moving with others helps the individual move through these emotions. Intense or negative feelings may emerge, but they permit the group to discuss old emotions as well as current ones. At one retirement home, for example, the movement activity I led prompted the group to discuss death. The activities described here are intended to motivate the group to release pent-up emotions.

In one of the groups I work with, a laughing movement performed by one woman sparked waves of contagious, invigorating laughter. When I asked the members of the class to express their feelings, they told me, "We feel happy." "Laughing relaxes you, it releases tension." "When I laugh, I cry and it seems to rinse and cleanse the whole body. It washes away my sadness." "It helps you forget your problems." "It's contagious and cheers you up."

Matching Motions with Emotions

To get a group started thinking about emotions, the facilitator asks the group to discuss some emotions that are shown on television or in movies. The facilitator may want to share personal emotional experiences with the group, and to ask other group members to share emotions they have experienced.

Next, the facilitator asks the group to create movements that reflect a particular emotion. Each member of the group thinks of an emotion (e.g., joy, anger, frustration) and then creates an appropriate movement (Figure 7). After each person displays a movement, the entire group imitates the movement so that each person in the group experiences the same emotion. Each movement should be repeated several times. For example, to reflect anger, the first person in the group might shake her fists. Everyone in the group would then imitate the fist-shaking movement. The next person in the circle would continue with

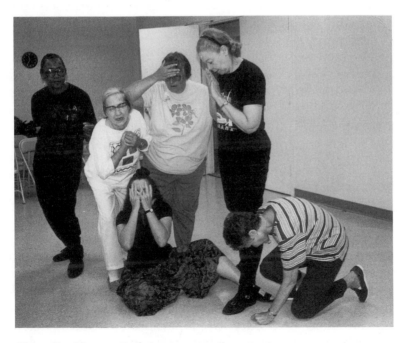

Figure 7.   Movements that express emotion.

the same emotion, perhaps by stomping her feet. After everyone repeated this movement, the next person might pound his fist down on his thigh and shout "No!"

By putting all of the movements together, the group creates a dance. The composition of the dance can be changed in a variety of ways. Sometimes the group has ideas on ways to modify a dance. The facilitator can also suggest ideas. For example, the tempo of the dance can be changed. A group can build a dance around the emotion of anger by beginning with quick angry movements, and gradually moving toward slower angry movements. Or, a dance based on joy can begin with slow joyful movements that increase in speed with each successive repetition.

Another good way to structure a dance is to have three different movements representing the same emotions done simultaneously by groups of three or four people. Adding props and costumes or costume touches, such as scarves, ribbons, or masks, enhances the intensity of the dance. Masks can be made by the group as a project, or a high school art class could be invited to design and make masks for the group as part of an intergenerational project.

The facilitator should remind the group that feelings may emerge as they perform their movements. Occasionally, intense feelings are expressed during this exercise, and group facilitators should be prepared to comfort participants. A movement facilitator does not have to be a therapist, but it helps to feel comfortable dealing with other people's feelings. Facilitators should allow the tears to flow and be available to comfort participants if necessary.

STORY DANCES

Dances can be used to tell stories. The stories may be based on past experiences or they can be made up as the dance proceeds. One way of beginning a story dance is to ask the group to take the experiences shared during the discussion of specific emotions and make up a story based on those emotions. Alternatively, a poem, short story, or fairy tale can be used as the basis of a story dance.

Story dances allow a group to bring in elements from other arts, including music, drama, visual arts, costume making, and poetry.

HAND DANCES WITH PARTNERS

In this activity, individuals in the group learn to relate to one another in a more intimate manner. The activity provides an opportunity for good eye contact and physical closeness.

Set up the chairs in two facing rows, about 2 feet apart from one another. Have each person pick a partner and sit down opposite the partner. Ask the group members to hold out their hands so that their palms touch their partners' palms, fingers facing up. Ask them to close their eyes and breathe deeply, concentrating on the warmth they feel from their partners' hands. After about a minute, have the group members open their eyes and allow their hands to separate from their partners' hands just enough so that their hands are no longer touching. Make sure that they hold their hands close enough together that the warmth is maintained between the two partners. Ask the pairs to move their hands apart a bit more, to the point where they no longer feel their partners' body warmth.

Next, ask the group to find ways to say hello with their hands (e.g., by waving, patting the hand, shaking hands) (Figure 8). Ask them to try to get to know each other better by studying each other's hands—variations in color, blemishes, veins, scars, and other marks that distinguish a person's hands.

After each person has become familiar with his or her partner's hands, ask the pairs of partners to try to use their hands to dance with their partners' hands, as if they were puppets on a stage. Hands can be together or apart during the dance. At some point, the facilitator should ask the participants to freeze, and to study the movements they had made. Throughout the dance, the group should refrain from talking.

When the group is ready to move on, the facilitator can suggest that they mimic the movements of fighting with their hands. Keeping physical safety in mind, participants should put as much energy as possible into wrestling, pushing, pulling, and gripping each other's hands (Figure 9). Once again, the group should be asked to freeze their movements, and to com-

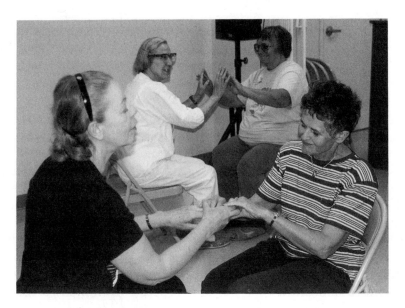

Figure 8.   Using hands to say hello.

pare how their body positions differed from their dance positions. Ask them to compare the emotions they felt during the
dance and fight sequences.

When the group is ready, the facilitator can ask them to
look for ways to use their hands to ask forgiveness and to say
farewell. As they let go of their partners' hands, they should
maintain eye contact for at least 10 seconds.

After this exercise is completed, ask the group to come
together to discuss the activity. Did they feel comfortable with
their partner right from the start? Did they feel closer to their
partner at the end of the activity? Did they find ways to say
hello using only their hands? What emotions did they experience during the mock fight?

Many people, particularly older women, find that they are
able to release repressed anger through this activity. Some people have difficulty with the fight sequence because they have
always avoided confrontation. This may be a good time to discuss confrontation. Because the activity involves physical contact, it is most appropriate for a group that has been meeting
together for some time and is comfortable with the facilitator

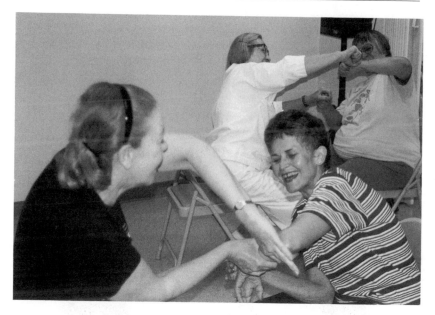

Figure 9.   A mock fight using hands.

and with each other. It is too physically demanding to be appropriate for frail older people.

CHARLESTON AND OTHER DANCES

Traditional dances, such as the Charleston, can be done both by people who can stand and people who cannot stand or who use wheelchairs. I have found that a group can have as much fun dancing in chairs as it can dancing standing up. I have taught the Charleston, the waltz, simple shuffle tap dances, and even the cancan to people who cannot stand up. I have also used line dances, such as the bunny hop.

Participants who are willing and able to stand up do so (Figure 10). For those people who remain in their chairs, I come and dance with each of them. I stand and hold their hands as we dance, letting them experience the flow of the movement and music. The movement brings a glow to their faces, and often the rest of their bodies sway in rhythm to the music. You can feel them dancing inside their bodies. They are dancing!

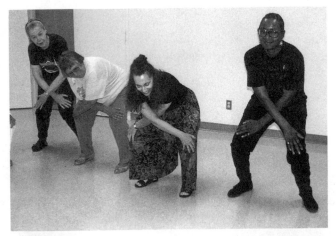

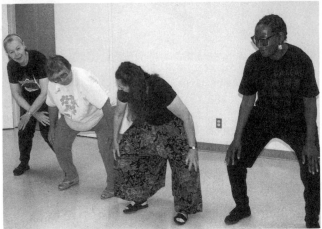

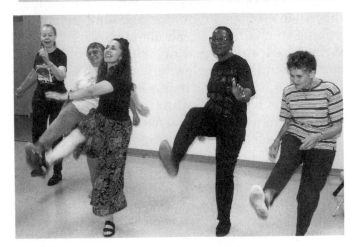

Figure 10.   Participants dance the Charleston.

During a demonstration in a group at a retirement home, a very frail woman said, "I can't move." I assured her that she could move and asked if I could move with her. With her permission, I took her arms gently and we moved together while she remained in her chair. Slowly, our arms made larger and larger movements. A smile came to her face and she obviously enjoyed the sense of moving safely. With very frail people, I may end my session dancing with each person in this manner. It may be anything from a polka to a cha-cha or a waltz. This gives us the chance for eye contact, personal contact, touch, and a shared movement experience, as well as a feeling of closure to the session.

Chapter 5

Movement Motivators and Props

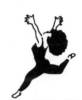

Angels can fly because they take themselves lightly.
—Scottish saying (from *A Book of Angels,* by Sophy Burnham)

Props are fun; they add a new dimension to exercise. While using some props, one resident at a nursing home said, "You get the fun out of us." A prop works as a focus outside of the self, motivating movement because of interest in the prop. I use a variety of props: some as motivators, such as scarves and bells, and some as tools for understanding the body and how it can move, such as a skeleton. Another way in which I use props is to help initiate creativity and new ideas, such as with pipe cleaners. Popping faces and sponge balls are wonderful motivators for squeezing the hands tightly in an isometric exercise that, if done often, can strengthen the hands and arms.

BALLOONS

Catch and Toss

For the very frail as well as the fit older adult, it is fun to catch and throw a balloon. They are light and fairly easy to catch, although sometimes they can be rather evasive. This also gives each person the opportunity to work one-on-one with the facilitator. After each has had a chance to catch and throw the balloon three times, I then ask them to hit it to me three times by either slapping or punching it. Some confused individuals may be able to do just one or the other (catch or hit). Any response is acceptable because it means an attempt is being made to pay attention and to participate. When working with anyone who has cognitive impairment, I attempt to reach or include them in whatever way I can.

In one nursing home, there was a woman who never responded to anything. She seemed to live in her own world. She was brought to the group each time in her wheelchair. During our introductions with musical instruments, I would play for her and say her name. One day when we were doing balloon tosses, I took the chance of tossing it to her after asking her if she'd like to catch it, not expecting to get a response to the question. Much to my surprise, she caught it. It may have been an automatic response, but it was a response. After that I became aware of her apparent attention (her gaze and head turn) during other activities as well.

Kick the Balloon

Give all participants a balloon and a Magic Marker and let them put their name, a design, or a mark of their own on the balloon.

For the very frail or those with cognitive impairment, the balloon may be placed at each person's feet to be kicked a few times with each foot. They also may attempt to kick it up in the air or to another person. For the fit, it is fun to stand in a circle and kick the balloon to another person, even using more than one balloon to build the excitement. In a mixed group in which there are some who cannot stand easily—or at all— those who stand form the circle with those in chairs included among them.

Another variation for a fit group, up to 10 at a time, is to make a standing circle and try to keep one or more balloons in the air, first with just hands and then with other body parts hitting the balloon. I usually begin with one balloon and add others, one at a time, until there are four or five balloons. This activity generates a lot of positive energy and motivates much movement and laughter. This activity can be done with persons who use wheelchairs, but it takes a lot more arranging and work to move all the wheelchairs and retrieve the balloons that fall out of the circle. One solution is to tie a string to each balloon and attach the balloons to five wheelchairs so they can easily be retrieved.

SCARVES

Using flowing musical accompaniment, such as a waltz, have each participant choose a lightweight, colorful scarf and hold it by one corner. The facilitator can have the group form a circle, standing or sitting, and make the following suggestions:

1. Reach the scarf as high and low as you can. (Repeat each movement a few times and repeat each with the other arm for those who can; for those who can't, repeat with same arm.)
2. Swing your arm in an arc, front and forward to the floor in front of you, then to the back and up behind you. Try to touch the floor with the scarf as you swing both forward and backward (Figure 11). For those who are standing, as you swing forward with your right arm, bend the knee of the forward leg and bend the torso in toward the center of the circle. As you swing up behind you, step out away from the circle, bending the knee again. Bring the circle of people close together so that the scarves create a colorful effect as they touch the ground.
3. For those who can turn around with the scarf, hold your arm out and let it flow in space in front of you. Turn to the right a few times and then to the left, so you can experience both directions. (If the facilitator and an aide have the energy, and it is appropriate, you can spin or turn persons who are in wheelchairs around so that those who cannot stand can still feel the sensation of spinning and the experience of seeing the scarf follow. Turn them to the right and then the left, so they can experience both directions.)
4. Wave the scarf from side to side, as far to either side as you can.

5. Circle the scarf around behind your head two or three times in one direction and then in the other. (This may be difficult for some because it takes coordination and a bit of physical ability.)
6. Make a big circle with the scarf, framing your whole body first in one direction, and then in the other, with each arm.
7. Wave and wiggle the scarf wherever you would like, perhaps trying to get it under your leg.
8. Have the scarf go over your head and under your body.

Ask for other suggestions from the group. You can also ask them to throw the scarf in the air and catch it with both hands, then toss it from one hand to the other. This is good for hand–eye coordination. Participants can have a game of catch (Figure 12) with a partner, each throwing his or her scarf at the other at the same time, so that they are catching their partners' scarves while the partners are catching theirs. With frail people, I throw my scarf to them at the same time they throw theirs to me, working with each person one at a time.

Have the group create their own scarf dance, moving the scarf any way they want. The facilitator may add more scarves to this activity at this point, so that the participants can have a

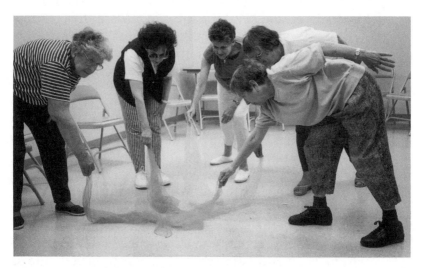

Figure 11. Bending and reaching to touch scarves to the floor.

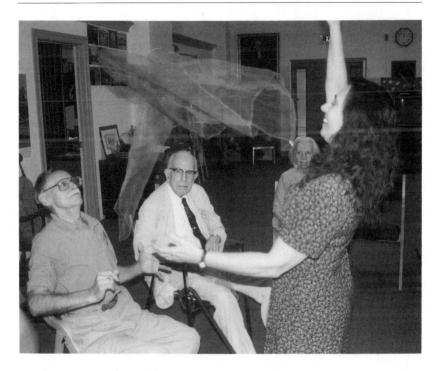

Figure 12.   Playing a game of catch.

scarf in each hand, or even playfully dress up with some around their hands, necks, waists, or wherever they wish. This activity can end with each participant using the scarf in a charade, as something other than what it is, such as a headband, a mask, an apron, or a tie, while the rest of the group guesses.

During the scarf activity at a nursing home, one inhibited lady, who said she considered herself clumsy, got up and danced. One man with very poor vision who was usually very hard to motivate got carried away with the scarf and didn't want to part with it.

Ask everyone to drop the scarf from high up and see how it floats. Then ask them to lift an arm and have it float down like the scarf did. For very fit people, you can ask them to float their whole bodies down to the floor and land in a shape like the scarf. Those in a chair can do this with their upper bodies, raising their arms and floating down as close to their legs as they can.

The scarves can also be used as a tool for color and environmental awareness. Ask each person what else in the room is the same color as his or her scarf. Or, ask the participants to hold their scarves up to their faces and look through the scarves to see how the hue of everything else in the room changes.

Two-foot strips of colorful crepe paper streamers can be used in place of scarves. They float just as easily and can be made into creative articles to be worn and kept by the participants, such as a bracelet, a bow for the hair, or a necktie.

BELLS ON ANKLES AND WRISTS

I have always enjoyed bells. I made some ankle and other body bells in the past when working with children at a summer camp, using jingle bells threaded through elastic. There were sets for wrists, ankles, heads, and waists. But I never thought of using this idea with older adults. I bought a set of ankle bells used by professional ethnic dancers and brought them into class one day, thinking I'd use them as an instrument to shake and pass around. But when I got to class, I decided to use them as an activity.

Let each person tie the bells around his or her ankles (giving help to those who need it). Anyone wearing stockings may tie them around his or her wrists so they won't tear the stockings. Let each person have a turn dancing with them, leading the rest in whatever movement he or she feels like, or whatever movement the bells stimulate. Each person can have the opportunity to dance alone for a while before the rest join in—it is a chance to solo. Those who cannot stand can move their feet, legs, and arms in their chairs.

I find this a wonderful motivator for all populations, including very frail people. Even those who rarely stand sometimes do so. The bells can be used on the arms as well, which motivates greater arm movements. I use African or Caribbean drum music to accompany the dancing. The sound of the bells as one moves promotes additional excitement and therefore more movement. Even those persons with diminished hearing are able to feel the vibrations of the bells. This activity also provides the chance to talk about other cultures that use bells as part of their traditional dances.

ELASTIC

Chinese jump ropes (Figure 13) can be used as initiators for creative movement. Group members individually explore what they can do, placing their feet on one end and their hands around the other end, stretching, twisting, and bending the arms, legs, and torso. After the group has the chance to find a variety of positions, poses, and movements with the elastic,

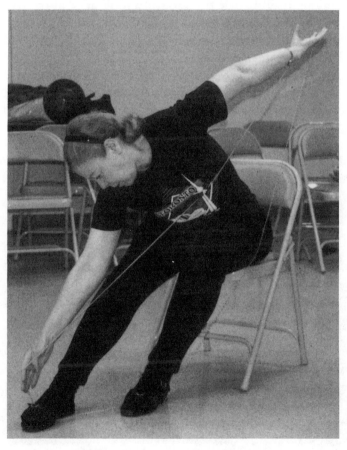

Figure 13.   Exploring shapes with a Chinese jump rope.

each member can find a shape to share that everyone can mirror, giving everyone the opportunity to lead in turn. This can be done in a sitting or standing position.

A variation of this would be for the group to partner up and have the partners tie their ropes together, exploring the shapes they can make together.

SKELETON

A 12-inch plastic skeleton (Figure 14) from a toy store can be brought to class and passed around so that participants can see the parts of the body I often mention. (Pictures of a skeleton also may be used.) I ask the group to look at, and try to move, the joints that bend, the rib cage, the pelvis, the hip sockets, and the vertebrae. I never pretend to be presenting an anatomy lesson, but the more we know about ourselves, the easier it is to understand how to take care of ourselves, and the more knowledge we have about our bodies, the easier it is to take responsibility for ourselves. I find that bringing in the skeleton not only gives information, but is fun as well. Many jokes emerge.

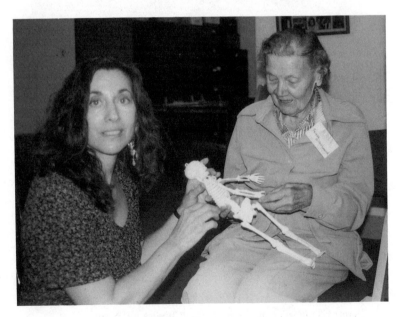

Figure 14.   Using a skeleton to study joints.

After seeing and feeling the skeleton, it is easier to feel those parts on ourselves as we move. For example, the group can partner up and take turns running their fingers down their partners' spines, feeling the vertebrae. The next time they are performing an activity involving rolling down or up the spine, "vertebra by vertebra" is more clearly understood. This examination of the skeleton can be repeated periodically, especially when presenting hands-on activities (see section on The Importance of Touch in Chapter 8). I have found that even very frail persons are able to better articulate their movements after examining the model skeleton.

PUPPETS

Sometimes I bring my puppets to class and give each person the opportunity to choose one. Then I ask them to introduce themselves to their puppets. I ask them to get to know their puppets, to have a conversation (Figure 15) with them, and to

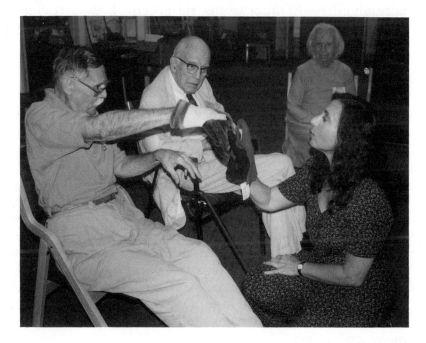

Figure 15.   A conversation with puppets.

listen closely to what their puppets say to them. This activity has worked particularly well with frail and confused elderly persons.

Some of the statements that were made by puppets are: "You're not very good-looking, but you're good, and when I ask you to do something you do it from your heart." "When you get ready he'll do anything." "Good morning, everybody, and I love everybody." "You can do it if you try." In one case, a woman in the geriatric unit of a hospital wouldn't take her medication, but, when the puppet asked her to, she did.

I also have had groups partner up and have their puppets introduce each other and say something about how they felt. There are some group members who feel silly and uncomfortable with puppets, and they may participate by watching.

Body parts can be puppets also. For instance, an elbow can be one person's puppet while someone else's shoulder acts as a puppet. In this case, the person whose elbow was the puppet would talk and the person whose shoulder was the puppet would answer as if the shoulder were responding to the other person's elbow. In other words, the specific body part chosen becomes the puppet. This can be done verbally or it can just be a dance movement conversation with no words.

BIRD, POPPING FACE, AND SOFT SPONGE BALLS

I often browse through toy stores, gift shops, and variety stores; it's surprising how much can be found that can be used to help motivate movement. The bird works to articulate gross motor movement in the arm and shoulder. Popping faces (Figure 16) are fun to watch and never fail to bring a smile to the person squeezing them, as well as to the rest of the group. As the popping faces are squeezed, the eyes, nose, and tongue pop out. After experiencing these in stress reduction workshops, many business people keep one on their desks to use as a stress reducer. Therapists can use them for stress reduction or as a tool for imaginative stories. These and soft sponge balls are good to help strengthen hands and lower arms when the person squeezes them. I encourage the older adults to squeeze hard and to do many repetitions.

PIPE CLEANERS

Colorful pipe cleaners also are good motivators. They are something that can be worked with outside of the body that helps to initiate bending and twisting shapes. After everyone has chosen a color, I ask that each person explore how many ways he or she can find to bend and twist the pipe cleaner, making a final shape to share with the group.

Each person has the opportunity to hold up his or her shape, and the rest of the group has the chance to move their bodies or a body part into as close an approximation as they can to each shape. In each group there are always interesting variations of shapes, ranging from abstract shapes to naturalistic shapes such as a flower, an animal, or an object, like an umbrella.

BEANBAG

I use beanbags to help with body part articulation, strength, and balance, and to have fun in the process. One of the beanbags I have looks like a mole. He has whiskers, is yellow with lovely eyes, a cute face, and velour skin, and is named Puggle. He lives in a blue velvet drawstring bag. The other one I have, whose name is Nuffling, has soft fur on top and velvet under him. He is heavier in weight than Puggle. Here are some ways in which I instruct those in the group to use whichever beanbag I pass around:

1. Place the beanbag on one shoulder at a time, first balancing it and then lifting the shoulder up three times. (For frail people, I do the placing. For persons with cognitive impairment, some of these activities help them to feel the body part and therefore make it easier to move it. The texture of the beanbag is a sensory experience as well.)
2. While sitting in your chair, place the beanbag on each thigh, balance it, and then lift the knee as high as you can three or more times, keeping the beanbag from falling. (The velvety underside of Nuffling sticks more easily and helps to keep him from falling. For very frail persons, lifting Nuffling's heavier weight is great exercise.)

3. Now balance the beanbag on your foot and lift the foot off (Figure 17) the floor as high as you can without dropping the beanbag. Do this a few times with each foot. (I go from chair to chair helping each person.)

4. Balance the beanbag on a body part (i.e., head, elbow held horizontally, or hand, palm up or down) and walk across the room. (I have had very creative variations on this activity from members of my classes. One woman placed Puggle on her back after she got down on her hands and knees, and then crawled across the floor. Another put the beanbag in her skirt pocket, while another placed it on his foot.)

5. Toss the beanbag up in the air three times and catch it with both hands, and then toss it from one hand to the other. Then try throwing and catching it with the same hand. (This is also good for hand-eye coordination.)

6. In a circle, have a catch with the person on your right, throwing the beanbag to the next person after a few catches.

7. Make a group circle standing up. First, call someone's name and throw the beanbag to that person. (This reinforces names and builds hand–eye coordination.) Next, quickly throw the beanbag to someone, who then has to do a body movement that everyone must imitate. (The beanbag is thrown by that person to another person, who does another body movement that the class follows, and so on until all have had a turn.) Finally, throw the beanbag to anyone of your choice. After that person catches the beanbag, everyone must bend down and touch the floor or do whatever movement you have designated. (Again, this activity is repeated until each person has had a turn to catch the beanbag.)

WORRY DOLLS

These are tiny dolls from Guatemala that come in a small box. The tradition is to take the doll from the box and give all your worries to this doll. I bring these dolls into all of my classes and find that everyone is able to silently give over their worries, after which there is a sense of release. I inform the class that I will place the worry dolls on my spiritual altar when I get home. After this ritual, the mood of the class is uplifted. We have shared in a ritual that is done with lightness and fun, yet it is effective.

OTHER PROPS

Teddy Bears

Included in my collection of props is a talking teddy bear, who repeats up to nine words. I pass him around and ask group members to describe what they like best about themselves. Sometimes I ask them to tell the bear what they are thankful for, or I may just say, "Tell the bear anything you like." This prop is special because participants get to hear their own words

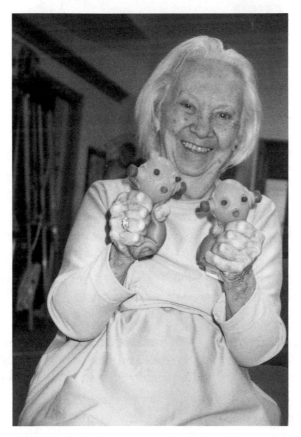

Figure 16. Popping faces motivate hand movement and stimulate laughter.

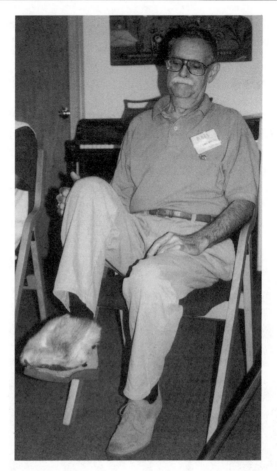

Figure 17.   A beanbag is used to help with body part articulation, strength, and balance.

repeated. I also have a bear who skates. After sharing him, we create a group skating dance or a sport dance.

Soft Dolls

I have a variety of colorful and fun soft dolls that I use to have a catch and toss with frail persons and persons with cognitive impairment. They are lightweight, easy to catch, and attract attention.

Rainbow Glasses

These are glasses that, when looked through and focused at either natural or artificial light, make beautiful rays of rainbows (Figure 18). I tell everyone that this reminds us that the rainbows are always there, it's just that we can't always see them. I had a friend whose father used to tell him to dust off his rainbows when he was depressed.

Streamers

I use these with both fit and frail persons. For group members who use wheelchairs, I have shortened the streamers by winding them around the handle, and I move each wheelchair into the center of the room so the streamers do not hit anyone. The bright and shiny streamers make wonderful designs as each person makes big circles (Figure 19) or other patterns using a large range of motion with first one arm and then the other.

Kaleidoscopes

These are great for initiating imagination and conversations by remembering other kaleidoscopes and other things the images

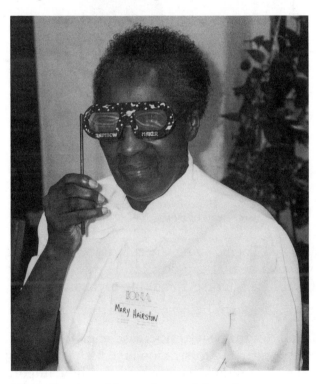

Figure 18.   A participant tries on rainbow glasses.

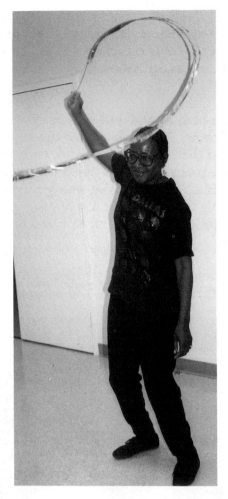

Figure 19. Moving a streamer uses a large range of motion.

remind you of. Poems about the colors and designs can be created, and each person can do a follow-the-leader movement that reflects his or her interpretation of the images.

Cookie Cans

An unusual yet fun way to increase energy and at the same time release anger and frustration is to kick the bottom part of a cookie can (the round shallow kind that hold imported cookies). Having an object outside of the self often serves as an excellent motivating force. The sound made as the can is being kicked adds another stimulating dimension. This also provides a good opportunity for venting some emotions. This activity is done by holding the can firmly in one hand, from a sitting position, from a standing position while holding onto the back of a chair for support, or while walking across a room, stepping and kicking one foot at a time. After everyone has had a turn, there are several variations on this I use when possible:

1. Standing next to your chair, and holding onto it when necessary, kick the can eight times, alternating legs.
2. Moving across the circle or the room, alternate step-kick, step-kick, eight times. (With those persons whose balance is questionable, but who want to try, I hold onto them.)
3. Holding the can in your right hand, behind you and down low, try to kick it from behind you with your left foot. (This requires coordination and concentration and often provokes laughter and giggles at the resulting confusion of body and mind.)

Be sure participants are wearing shoes that are not soft or opened toed, like sandals.

Kicking the cookie can is a great initiator for leg kicks. Very fit people can hold the cookie can in one hand as they reach out with the can, take a step, and kick as high as they can reach, followed by taking a step on the other leg and kicking with that leg, so that they are alternating kicking first with one and then the other leg, until they have taken eight steps and kicks. It is always a good idea to stand behind participants as they do this, prepared to catch them if they lose their balance.

People with insecure balance can hold onto the back of a chair with one hand and hold the cookie can in the other as they kick with alternating legs. Those persons who cannot stand or are afraid of losing their balance can do this in a sitting position. For frail people, I hold the can for them first over one foot, at a height appropriate for them, and then over the other until they have done eight kicks, alternating the leg they kick with so that one leg does not get too tired. Alternating is also better for coordination. For persons with cognitive impairment, I touch the knee of the leg to be lifted, and the sensory stimulation seems to help them understand what to do.

Chapter 6

Movement Games

You don't wake up one morning and say, "I will become a dancer." You wake up one morning and realize "I've been a dancer all my life," and you say to yourself "I am a dancer, I am a dance."

—Unknown

Movement games add structure to the exploration of body movement. They help to stimulate creativity and motivate body movement. They involve exploration of space, direction, perception, sensitivity, coordination, and touch, as well as fun and laughter. Most of the following activities are done in pairs or groups, which creates social interaction. These games work very well with Elderhostel groups or other physically able groups in senior recreation centers, retirement apartment complexes, and elsewhere. By varying some of these activities, they can be appropriate for a frail group as well.

MOVING TO AND FROM THE SELF

Open/close, widen/narrow, expand/contract, grow/shrink, and unfold/fold. These pairs of words help us explore various body parts and whole body movements when used in a game. Although the pairs of words are similar, each has a slightly different connotation, and the use of the body and muscles will change with each set of words.

Open/close (or pull in and pull out) has a quality of reaching out into the environment and coming back to the self, an out-and-in feeling.

Widen/narrow has an out-and-down, up-and-in quality. Widening includes a tendency toward squatting or bending. When narrowing, one may tend to go up on the toes to acquire a taller and thinner feeling and look—a sort of sucking in and lifting up.

Expand/contract may use the muscles by loosening and tightening, and may also have a more conscious awareness and use from the center of the body (chest, diaphragm, and pelvis).

Grow/shrink involves qualities that embody pulling into gravity, going in and down into the floor, or melting and then going upward and outward. These might be done more slowly.

Unfold/fold has more of a piece-by-piece (body part–by–body part) feeling and quality to it.

Each pair of words may initiate a different kind of feeling as well as a different way of moving for each person. Therefore, it is a good idea to try them all and then have a discussion about how the movement quality of each person differed for each set of words.

Start with the first pair of words, "open/close," and ask the group to explore each word by first opening and then closing the eyes, mouth, hands, arms, chest, and legs, one body part at a time. Those people who are able can open and close the whole body. This can be done on different levels and in different directions (i.e., up, down, side).

An example of opening and closing the whole body (Figure 20) to the side would be opening the arms and legs as wide as possible to the side, and perhaps even toward the back, allowing the head to lift upward, the chest to expand forward, and the back to arch. When closing the whole body, the legs could fold by bending at the knees and squatting; the chest could curve inward, with the arms folding into the chest; and the head could bend down, chin toward the chest. Those persons who are frail or are unable to stand can reach out as far to the side with as much of the body as possible, perhaps with just the arms going out and the chin reaching up, and then close inward by crossing the arms across the chest and allowing the head to drop down, chin toward chest.

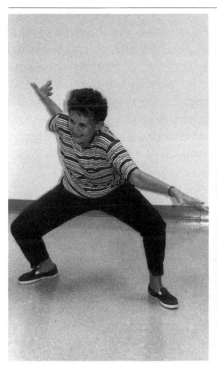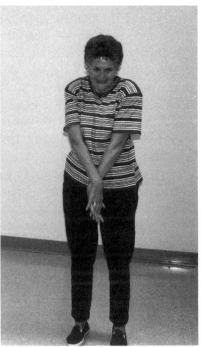

Figure 20.   Examples of opening and closing the body.

After exploring each of these sets individually, the group can pair up and try them with partners facing each other and perhaps holding hands. This may be followed by small groups in circular or cluster formations.

Here are some other words that you may want to add to this list: spread, shorten, enlarge, extend, increase, decrease, swell, wane, condense, stretch, inflate, reduce, melt, vanish, ebb, decline, diminish, shrivel, tighten, cramp, collapse, compact, wither, draw in, and crumble.

MIRRORING, TRIANGLES, AND DIAMONDS

Mirroring

The next set of movement games can begin with mirroring, a follow-the-leader activity. Each member of the group gets the chance to stand or sit in front of the group and do movements that the rest of the group follow. It is a good idea to remind the group that the person leading must move very slowly so that everyone can follow. The challenge is for the group to mirror the leader's movements, trying to move at exactly the same moment the leader does. Ask the person who is leading to make sure that his or her movements are always visible to the others in the group. For example, if the leader places his or her head and eyes down, the others in the group will not be able to see because, by following, they will also have their heads and eyes down.

Although this activity can be done in a circle, it can get confusing as to which side of the body does the following. When performed in a circle, it is easier to give the lead to the person on the right. When one leader finishes, he or she turns to the next person and perhaps gestures, with the arm or head, "*Your* turn."

In this activity, everyone has the opportunity to lead. For most people, mirroring is a fun experience. However, there may be a few participants who feel intimidated by leading, and freeze up. A person who doesn't know what to do can pass the lead on to the next person. No one should be forced into leading. Allow this to be a pleasant experience rather than a tension-producing or fearful one.

After the group has done this activity for a round or two and understands the concept, then it can be done in pairs, in a sitting or standing position. Ask everyone to find a partner. Both partners hold their hands up to each others' hands, fingers up, palms facing but not touching. The facilitator can designate when one partner starts to lead and when to have the other partner take the lead, or each person can take over the lead at any time. The person leading can start either at the facilitator's suggestion or when the person leading feels ready. The "leading" partner moves one or more body parts in slow motion, starting with the hands and arms; the "following" partner mirrors the movements, as though looking in a mirror and seeing his or her reflection move (Figure 21). You should emphasize that each person must be very observant and sensitive to every move and change in his or her partner's body.

The leading partner can slowly add more and more body parts, until the whole body, or as much of it as is desired and comfortable, is moving. The person leading needs to be sensi-

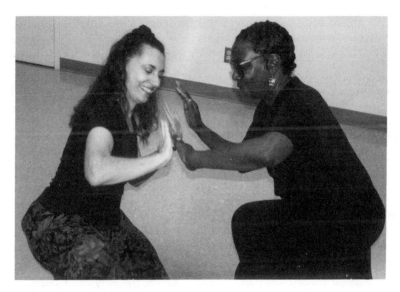

Figure 21. Mirroring movements.

tive to what his or her partner is capable of following and mirroring.

The facilitator can ask the group to freeze their positions
after they have been moving for a few minutes. While the
group is in these frozen statues, ask them to think about what
they might be doing, to imagine what these two statues are in
the midst of doing. Tell the group to remember their positions
and then to relax. Have each pair share ideas, first with each
other and then with the rest of the group. Each pair can demonstrate its positions to the rest of the class and share its ideas.

By changing the lead or changing partners completely, this
activity can continue for 10 minutes, or even longer. Changing
partners may change how each person moves because movement responses are different with different people. With a frail
group, the facilitator may have to move the chairs so that each
person has a partner facing him or her. The facilitator may also
want to lead the whole group rather than have the group work
in pairs.

Triangles and Diamonds

This variation of mirroring is good for use with uneven numbers of people and offers a chance to experience a wider range of

movement and movement personalities. This activity is suited to small groups of three and four and may not be appropriate for very frail persons. Standing approximately arm's-length apart, groups of three form the shape of a triangle and groups of four form the shape of a diamond. One person at a point of the triangle or diamond faces out and becomes the leader. The others face and follow the leader as he or she moves slowly. At first the movement should be made while the groups are standing in place, but after the groups have had the chance to become comfortable moving with each other, they may want to venture through space (taking the movement in any direction), as well as through another group.

For the leader to give up the lead, he or she must turn one way or the other and then face the person who becomes the new leader and is now the point of the triangle or diamond. In this way, the lead keeps changing while the shape of the triangle or diamond is maintained. Unless the facilitator signals otherwise, each leading person can move for as long or short a period as he or she desires. It is generally good to have a rule that everyone must turn to the right all the time, or else the same two people may find themselves exchanging the lead continuously.

Some followers will find that there are some leaders' movements that feel easy and comfortable and others that are difficult for their bodies. Some movements stretch them into pleasant new ways of moving, and others may be disliked. The group should be reminded beforehand not to do anything that is too difficult for others, such as a headstand or a cartwheel. (This is unlikely, but it can happen, particularly if the group includes someone who needs to prove his or her strength or who can do something difficult and wants to show it. There are also those who feel they want to challenge the group, or just make them laugh at an extreme movement that they know no one else will be able to follow.) The group also should be told to do the best they can when following and not to be concerned if they cannot do a movement exactly the same way as the leader.

This activity can also be frozen. Ask the group to freeze for a moment, at a point when the positions look interesting, and then ask them to look around while the rest of their bodies stay in these positions. This allows them to see the variety of movement and positions of the other groups. Then have them continue the activity.

It is nice to use background music that will not influence the movement; music that is slow moving and flowing, such as Kitaro's "Silk Road," would be appropriate.

PASSIVE/ACTIVE

In Partners

Ask everyone to find a partner. Have one member of each pair sit in a chair and relax as much as possible, letting the arms and legs go limp. This person is the passive partner. The active partner will first test how relaxed the other is by lifting his or her arm and asking the passive partner to go completely limp, like a rag doll, and to pretend that the arm weighs a ton. The active partner can lift the arm and let go of it to see if it will drop down. Some people cannot relax enough to do this, and their arms will remain in the air, or they will find themselves helping their partners. This can be practiced a few times. Sometimes it is just a matter of trusting another person with one's body—and that takes practice and time.

There are a number of different ways you can begin the activity. Tell the active person to proceed by placing the partner's body (arms, hands, heads, legs) in a pose that will form a sculpted creation. When everyone is finished, the active group can walk around the room to observe all the statues. You may even have each "sculptor" give a title to his or her masterpiece. Once the activity is completed, ask partners to switch roles and repeat the process.

This and the following activity may not be appropriate for a frail group for many reasons; for example, staying in one position might be too hard. However, with some creativity it may be able to be adapted for your specific group. For instance, the facilitator, after explaining the role of the passive person, could take the hands of a frail person, and lead him or her in very slow, gentle, and easy-flowing movement. The kinesthetic feeling (body sense) of being led and moving with another person can be a very satisfying experience. A frail person who has the energy or ability may enjoy taking another person's hand and leading him or her. Perhaps an aide can partner with a fragile person, who may enjoy gently pushing or pulling parts of the aide's body and watching as he or she responds in movement like a tree responding to the wind.

In Groups

Divide the group in half, asking one half to be "active" and the other half to be "passive." Quiet music, such as a lullaby or Japanese koto music, can be used to set the mood. Ask all of the participants who choose to be in the passive group to sit in their chairs or on the floor in the center of the room while the active group makes a statue of the passive group, connecting each person by one body part or another. A statue is made by lifting a passive person's arm or leg and having it connect to or rest on the body part of another person in the passive group. For example, an arm or leg of one person is held up by resting it on the shoulder or head of another, or the back of one person is leaned on the shoulder or leg of another. The group should be advised to be careful how they place the body parts, and to make sure the position will not cause injuries.

An important aspect of this game is that anyone in the passive group can at any time become active. This causes a constantly changing statue as well as changing groups, because anyone in the active group also can decide at any time to become passive. The facilitator may need to make sure that there is always a sufficient number of people in each group. The game may end at any time.

FILL-INS

Ask one person to start this movement game by making a body shape in the center of the circle. Then have the next person fill in this shape by either getting underneath the first person or in some way covering that person by placing his or her own body in a shape on top, but without touching, so that the first person can move away. When the first person has moved, another member of the group fills in the second person's body shape, after which the second person moves out of the shape, and so on. One at a time, each person in the class has a turn.

A second variation is to do this in pairs. The first pair makes a fill-in shape that a second pair fills in and so on until each pair has done it.

In another variation, the group can be divided into small groups of five or six. One group at a time can make a group shape that the next group can fill in until all the groups have had a turn both making a shape and filling in a shape.

This is not an appropriate activity for frail participants, but an alternative fill-in activity can be created. For example, each person can try to fill in a part of him- or herself by making a shape with one arm and placing the other arm inside it. Another way this can be varied is to have objects that can be filled in with a body part shape, such as making a shape with two arms or hands inside a hula hoop that is held by another person.

DRUM UP ENERGY

A great body part warm-up and picker-upper I use is to play a tape of a very upbeat drum solo. Music such as "Drums of Passion," or "Healing Session with Babatunde Olutunji," or drum solos by Mickey Hart are good for a more active group. A drum solo by Gene Krupa or perhaps a slower rhythm, such as some Latin music, might be more appropriate for a frail group. I begin this activity by showing my "drum bear." This is a mechanical toy bear that blows a whistle and then plays a drum. While showing this around the room, and getting smiles from everyone, I explain that as a child I had no toys and now I have many toys. After sharing Drum Bear, I announce that now we are all going to play on an imaginary set of drums. I ask those who can stand to do so and those who can't to participate while sitting. Once the music is playing, I instruct the participants to play their imaginary drums. I participate in all activities. After we have gotten moving, I tell the group to play their drums with their heads, and then their shoulders, followed by their elbows, chests, hips, and feet. I wait until they have had a little time for drumming with each body part before going on to the next one. Then I say, "You also have a set of drums underneath you and you have to bend low to play them." Next I say, "You have drums on either side of you, play them with different body parts. And now play the drums that are behind you, twisting your spine to reach as far as you can behind you on both sides. There is also a set of drums on the ceiling, let's kick them." Then I say, "Play all your drums with as many body parts as you can. Now play everybody else's drums; for those who can, move around the room." When I have a class who use wheelchairs, I tell them to play the drums of their neighbors on either side of them. I also go around the room playing everyone's drums.

This is a very high-energy activity and, when done with a great deal of enthusiasm by the participants, produces a contagious energy level that encourages everyone to join in the fun. Even very frail people are often motivated to move by a high-energy activity.

TISSUE GAME

This movement game takes concentration, coordination, and sensitivity. Give everyone a tissue (a scarf can be used instead) and ask each participant to place a corner of it in his or her right hand. Have the group choose partners and tell them to hold the other end of their partners' tissues in their left hands. Have each pair decide who will begin and, at a signal, ask them to begin a discussion with their partners. The subject of discussion can be anything they wish—sharing what they did the day before, telling a story about a family member or a friend, talking about what they like to do best, or expressing an opinion about an issue in the news. At the same time, both should be moving up and down, as well as under or over the tissue. They should move any way they can while continuing to talk and to hold onto the tissue without tearing it. If the tissue does tear, another can be taken. While this is easier to do with a scarf or a crepe paper streamer, by using a tissue, they must take more care in moving and pay more attention to their partners' movement as well as to their own.

A variation of this game is having the partners join another pair so that there are groups of four in a circle. You can arrange a group of six if there is a pair left over. Each person takes hold of the tissues held by the person on each side, and the group begins conversing and moving. Ask one person at a time to begin at a given signal. You also can tell the group to freeze at some point and then ask them to try to untangle without letting go of their tissues.

You may choose to make the game more complicated by having two groups of four join to make a group of eight. At this point, the conversations can be transformed into passing a sound from person to person while moving up and down, over and under, and all around.

As a conclusion to this game, ask everyone to make something creative with his or her tissue. Then have each person show his or her "masterpiece" and perhaps tell the group what it is and what it is for. It never ceases to amaze me that, just when I think I've seen everything that can be made with a tissue, no matter how many times I've done this, there are always at least one or two new surprises that result each time.

Chapter 7

Creative Fitness: Chair and Standing Exercises

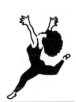

Common sense tells us that you've got to keep active to keep alive.

—Ossie Davis

S tudy after study has shown that exercise extends life— and improves quality of life. A recent study by Tufts University researchers showed that loss of muscle mass that occurs with aging can be partially reversed through exercise. Using weights with frail, institutionalized men and women age 90 and over resulted in significant improvement in strength and muscle mass (Fiatarone et al., 1994). Exercise stimulates the production of endorphins in the brain, which tend to elevate mood and increase tolerance to pain. Stretching the body also relaxes the brain.

A physical fitness class includes exercise for articulation of joints, flexibility, balance, and strength. Because exercise increases the respiration rate, it increases the supply of oxygen to the brain, which, in turn, serves to maintain mental alertness in the aging adult. After seeing photos taken during a More than Movement class, a staff member at a retirement home where I worked commented, "It is so nice to see the residents looking so alert; usually they aren't."

When facilitating a class focused on fitness I design my classes so that fitness is fun. It is a good idea to remind everyone: "Always listen to your own body; it is your best teacher. Do not do anything that gives you pain, no matter what I or anyone else tells you. Find your own limits." In my classes, I use both structured and unstructured activities. This chapter describes some of the structured exercises I use in my classes. Step-by-step instructions are provided for each one.

SITTING EXERCISES

Head

Before and during each exercise, remind everyone to keep breathing deeply. There is a tendency to hold the breath when concentrating, which can be dangerous during exercise. This exercise stretches the head and neck muscles, improving flexibility and strength.

- Slowly and gently bring your chin down as far as you can and as close to the chest as possible, then lift your head up, focusing your eyes to the ceiling. Repeat this four times.
- Now let your ear drop toward first one shoulder and then the other, being careful not to lift your shoulders. Gently stretch your neck from side to side as if you have heavy earrings in your ears. Repeat four times.
- Now circle your head four times to one side and four times to the other side. Imagine your nose or your chin drawing as large a circle as possible in the air. Or, imagine drawing a beam of light around in an enormous circle. You may hear a sound like Rice Krispies as you hear your neck snap, crackle, and pop. If head circling makes you dizzy, keeping your eyes open while circling may alleviate this.

There is some controversy about the safety of making complete circles with the head. It is my belief that each person needs to feel this out for himself or herself. Tell the class, "Remember, you are your *own* teacher—the teacher leading the class is only a guide whom you do *not* have to follow. Learn to pay close attention to what your own body tells you." To be safe, you may want to suggest that the class only move their heads from side to side, making half circles.

For those persons with cognitive impairment, you may want to use something visual to stimulate movement up, down, and side to side—perhaps a colorful doll, held high, then held low, and then moved side to side to attract attention. Or you may consider very gently holding the person's head in your hands and generating movement in these directions.

Shoulders

This exercise helps to loosen tension and strengthen muscles.

- Lift your shoulders up as high as you can and press them down as far as you can, twice. Stretch them forward and backward twice.
- Now place your hands on your shoulders and put your elbows out to the side trying to touch the elbows together in the front (Figure 22). Then stretch them back as far as possible. Do this twice slowly and four times quickly.
- With your hands still on your shoulders, aim your elbows out to the side and move them up and down four times slowly and four times quickly, as if you were a bird flying. Now draw large circles in the air with the elbows four times in one direction and four times in the opposite direction.
- Keeping your hands on your shoulders, now try to place both elbows first on one leg and then on the other (Figure 23), stretching and twisting the spine. Aim to reach as close to your hip as you can and do this four times to each side.

For persons with cognitive impairment, placing your hand or a beanbag on the shoulder to awaken the tactile sense may help to initiate movement. Or, you may actually gently (never force any movement) lift the shoulder with your hands.

Fingers and Hands

This exercise helps to alleviate tightness in the joints caused by arthritis.

- Stretch your fingers out as wide as you can. Make tight fists; shake them like pepper shakers and throw them away, stretching your fingers out as you do so. Repeat four times.
- Now wiggle all your fingers as if you were playing a piano; now wiggle them like you are typing or playing a banjo. (You might ask the group to suggest other things they do that get the fingers moving and stretched.)

- Keep wiggling the fingers as you reach up high above your head, under your chair, or as close to the floor as you can. Wiggle the fingers of both hands first on one side of your chair and then on the other side, then behind your neck, and then behind your back.
- Keep wiggling the fingers as you stretch your arms open wide, then cross them over your chest and give yourself a hug, because you deserve one.
- With both hands, at the same time touch one finger at a time to the thumbs of the same hands—first your pointing fingers, then your middle fingers, next your ring fingers, and last your little fingers. Repeat this process four to six times, doing it a little faster each time. (This takes some coordination and articulation that is difficult for some.)
- Now shake out your hands and circle your wrists four times in each direction.

For persons with cognitive impairment, you may have to literally move the fingers gently to get some articulation. Or, you can try to find a creative object or prop that initiates finger

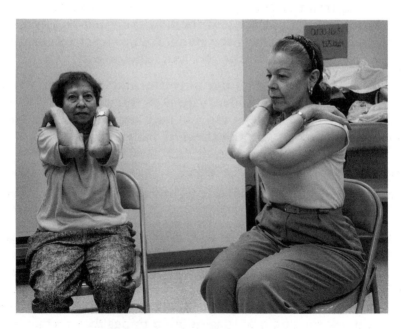

Figure 22. Participants practice shoulder exercises.

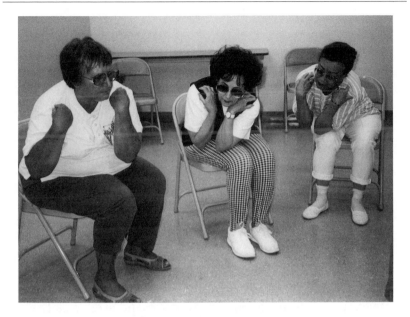

Figure 23. Twisting and stretching the spine.

manipulation and that might stimulate enough interest, such as a mini-piano that would also make a sound. However, initiating finger articulation may be difficult.

Side Stretches

This exercise makes use of the spine as well as stretching the sides of the torso.

- Hold onto your chair with your right arm and lift your left arm over your head, keeping it near your ear.
- Now take a deep breath and let it out as you reach over your head (Figure 24) like a rainbow or an arch toward your right side, reaching with a straight elbow toward your neighbor and stretching your torso (keep both buttocks on the chair).
- Now come back to center (upright spine), change arms, take a deep breath, and repeat to the other side. Continue changing sides until you have done three or four of these curved stretches to each side.

Any props that motivate larger arm movements in any direction would be appropriate for very frail persons.

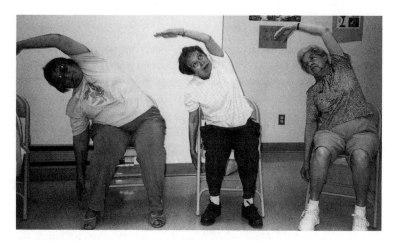

Figure 24.   Arm reaches stretch the side of the torso.

Reaching and Bending

This exercise strengthens the stomach and stretches the side muscles, helping to tone up the waistline.

- Reach up with both arms as high as you can, stretching the elbows as straight as you can, then reach down as low as you can, aiming to touch your toes or the floor. Do eight sets at a fairly quick pace.
- Then reach as up as far as you can to the left with both arms, and then try to touch the floor on your right side, doing four sets. (Some participants might get confused or not know their left from their right, so saying, "one side and then the other," may be more appropriate.) As you do this, imagine that you are reaching high up on a top shelf for a blanket or an old photo album, then placing it on the floor next to the chair.
- Reverse sides and repeat four sets of reaching up tall on one side and touching low on the other side.

Arm Exercises

These exercises are a fun and creative way to use the arms while extending the range of motion.

Swimming

For those who never learned how to swim, this can be like a swimming lesson. You can tell everyone to imagine that they are in a race across the English Channel. Jokingly remind them that it is much easier without water.

- Imitate swimming strokes. First do the crawl, reaching forward with each arm as far front as you can as well as reaching with the upper torso and turning the head as if you were swimming. Do this eight times.
- Next try the backstroke, letting the head and eyes follow each arm as it circles back. (In some facilities, the couches or the chairs do not permit this kind of movement.)
- Now try the butterfly stroke. Placing the backs of both hands together, palms out and thumbs down, reach both arms forward and out from the chest as far as you can before opening the arms out and around to the side; then start again. Repeat eight times. Use only one arm if you do not have use of both. (The butterfly stroke is another arm movement that uses both arms at the same time. Always remind those with limited use of their bodies to move whatever parts they can, because "what you don't use, you lose.")

Calisthenics

Other arm movements can include some basic calisthenics, such as:

- Place your hands on your shoulders, reach them up in the air, and then return them to the shoulders. Repeat this eight times.
- Then do eight sets of reaching out to the side and back in to the shoulders.
- Now reach down with the arms and return to the shoulders eight times.

Ballet Movements

I also like to include graceful balletlike arm movements using music such as waltzes.

- Opening your arms to the side, allow one arm at a time to reach over your head toward the other arm and back out again, with the torso following. Alternating arms, do this eight times.
- Repeat by reaching each arm across the body toward the other arm, letting the head and eyes follow the moving arm. Again, alternate arms and do eight times.

- Then swing both arms over the head from one side to the other like a willow tree, eight times.
- Next, starting on your right side, let both arms swing around front and to the left side, going from side to side, following the arms with the head and eyes.
- With your arms out one on each side, level with the shoulders, circle them down, crossing them as they lift, up and out to the side eight times, making the circle as big as you can. Then reverse the circle and end with the arms crossed on top of the legs.

This series of exercises makes use of the arms as much as does calisthenics, but gives a sense of rhythm, dance, and flow.

Churning Butter

This exercise is particularly good for those who cannot stand, but is beneficial for everyone. It gives them a chance to use their torso and hips.

- While holding onto a chair, use the image of churning butter as you make large circles with the torso, as if your head and torso were a stick.
- Try to lift each hip and buttock as the body moves around, reaching your chest as close to your legs as possible.

Standing and Sitting

This method of standing up makes use of gravity to make standing and sitting easier. It is also a good exercise in itself.

- Place one foot in front of the other; hold onto the sides of your chair and lean your body weight forward, letting gravity help you.
- Push your feet against the floor and your hands on the chair as you aim forward and up.
- Practice this process a few times, reversing it to sit.

STANDING EXERCISES

In a group with mixed abilities, for those persons who can't stand, offer an alternative exercise that can be done in a sitting position.

More Arm Exercises

These exercises help to maintain mobility of and circulation of the arms

- In a standing position, all facing the center of the circle, place your right arm forward, keeping the elbow straight. (For some persons, left/right differentiation is difficult, so you may use this to help increase awareness and memory, or you may just say, "Place one hand...")
- Slowly move your arm front, up, back, and then down as far as you can, making a large circle that starts from the shoulder, not the elbow. Slowly repeat this twice, a bit faster, and then eight times spinning your arms like a windmill or a propeller. Repeat with the left arm (other arm).
- Now turn sideways, so that you don't hit anyone when moving your arms. Reach your arms out to the side first, then circle them down, across, and up, twice slowly, twice a bit faster, and then eight times as fast as you can, circling your arms down, up, and around.
- Face center again. Lift your arms, bent at the elbows, chest high, pointing the fingers of both hands toward each other, palms down. Quickly pull the elbows back toward the shoulder blades, back of you, and release them back to starting position, eight times. (This develops the pectoral muscles on the upper chest.)

Push-ups Against a Wall

This exercise is good for the back of the upper arm (tricep muscle), the part of the arm that tends to get flabby.

- Place your hands on the wall, chest high, fingers facing each other. Make sure you do not lift your shoulders, and keep them as relaxed as possible. If it is too difficult to have the fingertips facing, then point your fingers toward the ceiling. Place your feet far enough away from the wall so that your body is leaning toward it at an angle.
- To a slow count of four, push smoothly away from the wall (Figure 25), and in a slow count of four come back, trying to touch your nose gently to the wall. Do not jerk or stop at each count. Be careful to move your body all at once so that

your pelvis is not sticking out. Take it with you as you move.

• Do this eight times, more or less, according to your strength and ability. If you need to, start with four and increase the number slowly over time. However, if you have the ability to do eight, do so and then rest, taking your arms off the wall and shaking them out. Then repeat another eight, taking one count to reach the wall and one count to push away from the wall until you have counted to 16, making another eight push-ups or push-offs.

For those persons who can't stand, have them place their hands together, chest high, elbows out to the sides, and press

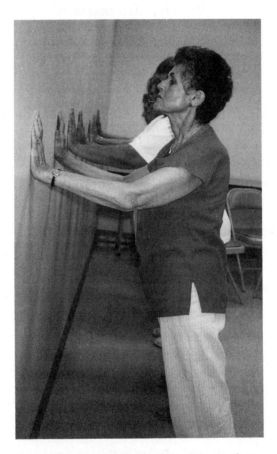

Figure 25.   Exercising triceps by doing push-ups or push-offs against a wall.

the hands together for eight counts and then release. Tell them to repeat this isometric exercise four to eight times.

Knee Bends and Metatarsal Stretches

This exercise is good for stretching calf muscles and the metatarsals, which are in the arches of your feet.

- If necessary, hold onto the back of your chair with one or two hands. Place feet about 6–12 inches apart, keeping your toes forward and feet parallel.
- Bend your knees, being careful to aim them directly over your toes. If you turn your knees in or too far out beyond the toes, you may injure them. Be aware of this whenever you bend your knees. Then straighten (without locking) your knees; repeat eight times. Be conscious of keeping your torso upright; avoid tilting forward.
- Now lift your heels off the ground, standing on the balls of your feet. Be careful not to turn your ankles. Move your body straight up, just as if a marionette string were attached to the top of your head and you were being lifted to the ceiling right above you. Do not lift your shoulders. Then lower your heels; repeat eight times.
- Now alternate bending and straightening your knees with lifting and lowering your heels, combining the two exercises. Try to do this smoothly without any jerks, as if you were moving through water. Do this exercise in a set of eight, trying to balance on the balls of your feet for a few moments at the end. If you are holding onto a chair, try to let go and maintain your balance.

Those participants who can't stand can lift their heels on and off the floor while their feet remain in a parallel position.

Torso Swings

This exercise assists in loosening the spine.

- Think of your spine as a maypole and your arms as the ribbons hanging from the maypole. As you bend your knees over your toes, swing your arms around your body as far to the side as you can, resulting in a gentle twist of the spine.
- Straighten your knees as you face forward and bend them again as your arms twist to the other side.

- Count a swing to both sides as one set and repeat each set eight times.

Arm Reaches and Back Rolls

This reaching and stretching exercise helps to stretch the entire body, as well as the hamstrings (the long muscles at the back of the legs) when rolling the head down to the floor and bending and stretching the knees. The rolling down and up helps improve articulated movement of the spine and torso. This exercise can be done from a standing or sitting position.

- Reach to the ceiling with both arms, as if you were picking apples off a very high tree branch. Other images to keep in mind might include climbing a ladder or a rope.
- Now reach both arms up and, with one arm at a time, stretch as high you can from the heels to your fingertips eight times, keeping the elbows straight.
- Then let your body melt down slowly, arms and head first, in a rolling manner, vertebra by vertebra, as far down to the floor as you can, aiming to touch your toes to the floor, head down.
- Remain in this position while you bend your knees and then straighten them twice. Then bend your knees once more and roll up your spine to a standing position, vertebra by vertebra.
- Repeat this series three more times. (If necessary, let the group do two sets and take a break by going on to the next activity before repeating the last two sets.)

Hips

This exercise helps to stretch several important muscles that provide for movement of the torso and legs. These muscles are attached to the top of the pelvis, in an area called the iliac crest. Most of us in this culture do not often isolate articulated movement of the pelvis. Fast disco music helps make this exercise fun.

- Imagine you have two strings tied to your waist, one on each side with a ball attached to each string at hip height. Hit the imaginary ball with your hip, on each side twice in a set of eight, and then hit each once alternating sides to the count of eight.

- Now make a complete circle with your hips in each direction as if you were using a hula hoop. (I have been told by some of my students that there used to be a dance step like this called Messin' Around.)
- This can be followed by making figure eights with the hips in both directions, or by writing your name with your pelvis. Don't forget to cross the "T's" and dot the "I's."

Legs and Feet

The exercise with the feet works the metatarsal and ankles, increasing flexibility and strength of the feet. The leg swings articulate movement for the hips and help to improve flexibility, strength, and balance.

- Stand behind your chair. Holding onto the chair back, open the feet out and stand with the legs far apart, heels lined up under your hips, and toes out comfortably. Bend one knee over the foot, keeping the heels down. Straighten that knee and then bend the other knee. One at a time, do this eight times. Be sure the knees bend out and over the toes. (This stretches the inner thigh, but may be difficult for some to do. Proper attention to knee alignment prevents injury. If the knee is turned in or out behind the toes, there will be a strain on the knee.)
- Next, bend both knees out at the same time, feeling that a marionette string is lifting your head and torso in the upward direction so that you don't sink, and then straighten your knees. Do this eight times. Stand close to your chair and be sure that your tailbone goes straight down so that your rear end is not pointing out and away from you. When you lift up, push your feet into the floor and feel the top of your head and your whole spine lifting toward the ceiling.
- Now bring your feet together, but keep the toes turned out without force, heels touching. Lift one heel off the floor, pressing into the ball of the foot, and then lower the heel. Do this four times on each foot.
- Follow this by pushing off the floor by rolling through the foot up to where only your toe is touching the floor, as you spring the foot off, pointing the toes downward and lifting the knee high on the side. Do this four times on each side and then repeat.

- With the toes pointing straight ahead, kick your right heel toward your buttocks, bending your knee, alternating four times on your right and four on your left, and then repeat.
- Making sure you are far from furniture or people, so that you have enough room, kick backward while keeping the leg straight. Alternate backward kicks, four right, four left, four right, and four left.
- Follow this by placing your left hand on the back of your chair and turning your body sideways, right arm out to the side. While maintaining weight and balance on your left leg (leg closest to the chair), point your right leg (leg furthest from the chair) behind you, ready to swing your right leg (outside leg) front and back. Allow your leg to brush the floor as if it were a broom, and swing loosely from your hip keeping your torso as upright as you can. Count one swing front and back as one set and do eight swings. Turn your body and repeat on the other side.

SITTING EXERCISES FOR THE LEGS AND BACK

General Exercises

These exercises help strengthen the psoas muscle, which flexes the thigh and assists in movement of the lower back.

- Bring a knee up to your chest and hug the knee with both hands as close to the chest as possible (Figure 26). Alternating legs, do a set of eight.
- Repeat the set of eight, this time aiming first your chin to each knee, then your nose, your forehead, and, finally, your right ear to your right knee and your left ear to your left knee. (This stretches the lower back and the back of the thighs.)
- Lifting and holding your leg from under the thigh and near the knee, extend your leg, stretching and straightening, as high as you can. Then lower the lower part of your leg, bending the leg from the knee, but keeping the thigh lifted. Extend and lower four times slowly, then increase the speed to a kick for four more sets. Change legs and repeat.
- Now change legs and still holding your leg from under the thigh extend the leg in the air, pointing the heel to the ceil-

ing, then the toes to the floor (flex and point). Do four on each leg, bending the knee after each flex and point.

- Then, to release any tension that may have built up, do a self-massage by using the heels of your hands to rub forward four times on each thigh, like a rolling pin. Then knead each thigh like dough and pat each like a bongo drum to stimulate the skin.
- Keeping both legs extended in the air straight out in front, point the toes down toward the floor and then back up toward your nose as far as you can. Do four sets slowly and four sets faster. Then point the toes inward toward each other and outward to the sides, letting the heels touch—four times in and out slowly, and four times in and out faster. (I sometimes say, "Let your toes kiss and let your heels kiss.")
- Now circle the feet so that the ankles are going through articulated movement. Imagine that you are drawing circles in the air with our toes, going four times in each direction.
- In chairs, march with your knees up high, doing four sets of eight.

Elbow-to-Knee Touch

This exercise can be done from a sitting or a standing position. Tell the participants to bring their right elbows and left knees together, twisting the spine (they should touch the elbow and knee if they can). Next, tell them to bring their left elbows and right knees together; have them alternate these movements eight times.

Bike Ride

Tell participants to start with the right leg and bring the knee up and push out front with the foot, making large circles just like riding a bicycle. When they have completed four circles in one direction, have then reverse the direction of the circle and do four more. Repeat with left leg.

Leg Lifts

This exercise was suggested to me by Mary Brewster, from a retired senior volunteer program, who assisted me in one of my classes. Ask participants to imagine that there is a milk carton placed on the floor at the right corner of their chairs. Tell them

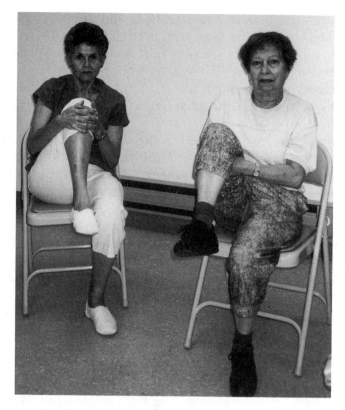

Figure 26.   Knee to chest exercise.

to lift the right knee high and bring the right leg over the carton and around to the right side of the chair, onto the floor, and then back over in front again, until they have done the entire movement eight times. Then have them repeat this with the left leg on the left side of the chair.

MAT AND FLOOR WORK

Getting Down on the Floor

Just getting down to the floor and back up again (Figure 27) is an exercise that is very important for the older adult, who may lose the ability to do many everyday things such as getting in and out of a tub or in and out of a car. With practice, the muscles required to get up and down can be strengthened, thereby providing more mobility.

- Begin by standing next to your chair. Reach for the floor with one hand and go down on one knee and then reach with the other hand and go down on the other knee.
- You may use your chair as a support if you wish. In that case, you may want to put one hand on the seat of your chair as a support while your other hand is reaching for the floor, and then place one knee on the floor, followed by the other hand and other knee.
- Now slowly sit on one hip, slide your arm and torso down to the floor, and roll over onto your back.

Some individuals will need to have a small pillow or a rolled towel placed under their heads.

Mat Exercises

For those persons who have mats or who are willing to use a large towel and who are able to get down on the floor, these exercises are very good for the lower back and spine. For those who have problems with their back, these exercises also can help to strengthen and stretch the back as well as strengthen the stomach. I have included a few leg exercises as well. Be-

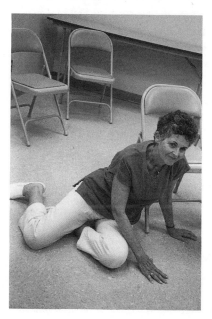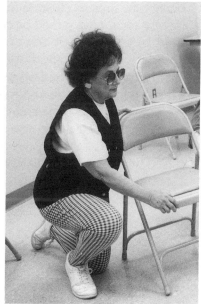

Figure 27.   Getting down on the floor.

cause there is less effort fighting gravity when you are lying down, it often is easier to work some parts of the body from this position.

There are times when some people may want to try these exercises but are afraid to. Offering help and encouragement may change their minds. Be sure that, if you offer help, you are strong enough to give support. If not, enlist the help of some other member of the group or staff. In some groups, only a few people will be wiling to try when you first begin floor work, but if you continue to offer the exercises, along with encouragement, more people will join in. For those persons who have had strokes or who have given up trying because of other injuries or pain, getting down and back up again not only builds self-confidence and self-esteem, but gives them the courage to try other things they thought they couldn't do. Be sure to give alternate exercises to those persons who decide not to, or can't, get down to the floor.

Pelvic Rocking

- On your back, put your feet on the floor as close to your buttocks as possible with your knees up. If you are on a mat, bring your hips as close to the edge of the mat as you can.
- Gently rock your pelvis back and forth, first moving toward your head and then toward your feet, trying to get your waistline closer to the floor, then relaxing and releasing it. Pushing with your feet helps.
- After doing this six to eight ties, gently roll your pelvis up off the floor vertebra by vertebra, as far as you can, in the direction of your shoulders (see Figure 28). Keep your feet and knees together so that you use more of your inner thigh muscles. Then roll down slowly, vertebra by vertebra, trying to place your waist down before your buttocks. Repeat four times.

Knee Hugs

- Bring your knee up to your chest and hug it with your hands at the same time that you raise your head toward your knee. Put your head down when you slide your foot forward, pressing your heel toward the wall in front of you. Repeat four times with each leg.

- Bring both knees up to your chest and hug them with your hands. Repeat four times, and on the fourth time gently rock from side to side, just on either side of your spine so that you do not roll all the way over on your side, feeling the massage you will get from the floor or mat. If you need to, you can stop yourself with your elbows so that you do not roll all the way over.
- Repeat this with your head reaching toward your knees, rolling from side to side after the fourth head reach.

Twisting and Stretching the Spine

- Placing your arms straight out, one on each side, bring both of your knees to your right side, trying to keep both shoulders down on the mat. Feel the stretch in your back.
- Keeping your elbow as straight as you can, move your left arm (opposite arm) in large counterclockwise circles, as close to the floor as you can, across your body and over your head, following your hand with your eyes. Do this four times going up and four times going down.
- Repeat to the other side, bringing your knees to the left side and circling with your right arm.

Sit-ups

This exercise is a modified sit-up that works the abdominal muscles to strengthen the stomach, thereby helping the back.

- Still on your back, knees up and feet on the floor, place your right ankle on top of your left knee, and let the right knee open to the side as much as you can.
- Slide your arms and hands forward, stretching toward your feet and slightly off the floor; raise your head and shoulders and hold them for 10 counts, and release back down to the floor slowly. If this hurts your neck, keep your chin up toward the ceiling rather than pointing it down into your chest.
- For those people who can't cross the legs, bend the knees and keep the feet on the floor close to your body and reach your hands toward your knees. It helps to breathe in slowly on the release and breathe out slowly as you reach forward.
- Do this four to eight times and then change legs and repeat on the other side.

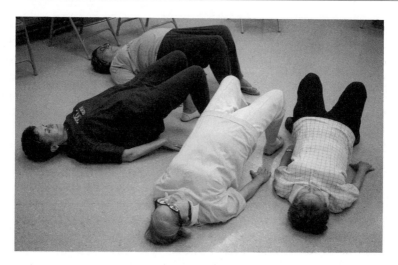

Figure 28.   Rolling pelvis up vertebra by vertebra.

Leg Lifts

Still on your back, with your feet on the floor and the knees bent, straighten your right leg on the floor. Do eight leg lifts at your own pace with your right leg, trying to keep your leg straight. Lift the leg as high as you can and place the whole leg on the floor after each leg lift. Repeat with the other leg.

- Roll over to your right side, supporting yourself with your left hand on the floor in front of you. If it is more comfortable, bend your right leg under you. Now do eight leg lifts with your left leg, pointing the knee toward the ceiling as it lifts and keeping the leg as straight as you can. Bend your knees and roll over to your left side and repeat this with your right leg.
- Roll over onto your hands and knees and come to a standing position, one foot at a time.

Moving Through Space

Using fast and upbeat music, have the group do four sets of eight fast walks around the room, going in any direction they please. Next, ask them to walk for eight counts, and then bend and touch the floor. Have the group do four sets of these. The object is to get everyone moving using both walks and bends. The facilitator also could make use of fast dancing or any of the creative movement activities that are relatively fast and fun.

PART II

MIND AND
BODY ACTIVITIES

Chapter 8

Relaxation, Imagery, and Touch

You cannot change the wind, but you can adjust the sails.
—Unknown

M any people have difficulty falling asleep. Sometimes we are anxious, in pain, or frustrated. Other negative feelings can also cause stress and tension. The following are a few techniques that are easily taught and learned. It must be remembered that, although tools can be readily acquired, if they are not practiced and used they can't do any good. It is each person's responsibility to give himself or herself permission to say, "Halt, stop," and to take a few minutes to do something to relax. It may be easier to pop a pill, but it is healthier to let your body and mind rest, and find physical and emotional calm by deep breathing, and by relaxing, using one of the methods described in this chapter. Additional suggestions on relaxation are provided in Chapter 11.

RELAXATION

Sometimes music helps us relax. If you decide to use music, choose gentle meditative music with no words. Environmental music, such as sounds of the ocean or a gurgling brook, is also appropriate. If you are in nature, listening to the natural sounds is ideal.

Whenever possible, it is best to do these exercises sitting in an upright position, with backs straight, feet uncrossed and placed on the floor, and hands gently resting on the lap. Suggest to the class that if they are wearing anything binding, such as a tight waistband, glasses, or jewelry, that they loosen or remove it.

Diaphragmatic Breathing

Natural breathing starts in the diaphragm and not in the chest. Place your hands on your stomach and diaphragm as you breathe, and feel the area expand like a bellows. Let go and soften your belly. If you watch an infant in a crib you will notice the breathing begins in the belly (the same is true of animals). Remember to soften the belly as you begin any of the following exercises.

Watching Your Breath

Either audiotape or read the following instructions *slowly, softly,* and *gently.* Allow a short pause after each sentence to give participants time to complete each suggestion.

> Close your eyes and concentrate on your breath. If you have difficulty keeping your eyes still while they are closed, try focusing on the bridge of your nose with your eyes closed. This helps to keep the eyes still. Focus on the area around your nose, slowly breathing in as deeply as you can, all the way down to your toes. Then slowly breathe out as far as you can, emptying your body of breath. Breathe in fully and breathe out fully. Breathe in and fill your body with breath, following your breath all the way in and all the way out. Notice the coolness of your breath as it enters your body, following it all the way in, and notice the warmth of your breath as it exits your body. Coolness in— warmth out; coolness in—warmth out.
>
> Become aware of any thoughts that enter your mind. Take note of them, but do not get attached to them. Let go of the thoughts as if they were puffs of smoke or clouds dissipating, or a wave in the ocean curling over and riding from the beach back out to sea.
>
> Bring your attention back to your breath, breathing in and breathing out. Remember that breath is the bridge to life. Breathe deeply. Take note of the split second of no breath, when you change from breathing in to breathing out, and see if you can hang there a couple of seconds longer. Now repeat this in the split second when there is no breath between breathing out and breathing in. Repeat both of these again.

Reentry

To bring the group back to an awakened state, read or audio-tape the following instructions. Remember to speak slowly, softly, and gently.

> Become conscious of how your feet are making contact with the floor and how your hands are making contact with your legs. Feel the weight of your hands on your lap. Just be aware; don't think about it. Pay attention to how your body is making contact with the chair. What parts of your body are touching the chair, and how? Are some parts of your body pressing or leaning, or do you feel as if the chair is holding you up? Take another deep breath and slowly become aware of those around you and the room you are in. And, when you are ready, open your eyes.

Once you have completed this relaxation exercise, ask for responses: "How do you feel? Were you able to relax?" One or two people may actually fall asleep; that's okay. Most will be very relaxed, quieted down, and not very talkative. Use this re-entry after each relaxation exercise.

Sets of Five

This method of relaxation has a different focus of concentration. Remember to speak slowly, softly, and gently. Read or audiotape the following instructions:

> Close your eyes and take a few very slow and deep breaths. Be aware of breathing in as far as you can—plus a little more—and then breathing out as far as you can—plus a little more. Now slowly and deeply breathe in through your nose and out through your nose, repeating this five times. You can keep count by touching the thumb of one hand to each finger of that hand in sequence, repeating as needed. Breathe as if there is a feather in front of your nose that you don't want to blow away.
>
> Now slowly and deeply breathe in through your nose and out through your mouth, repeating five times. Follow this with slow and deep breathing in through your mouth and out through your nose, again repeating five times. Finish this process with five slow and deep breaths in and out of your mouth.

Once you have completed this technique, bring the group back to an awakened state using the instructions for reentry, or in your own way.

This relaxation exercise can be done in sets of three, five, or seven. To enhance this relaxation exercise, the breathing sets can each be related to an element (earth, water, fire, and air) and a specific color connected to each. Tell the group to envision each element with its related color as they breathe. This helps them to focus on the breathing and to remember where they are within the exercise. It also provides a calming mental image. The following chart links elements and colors to each breathing set:

Element	In	Out	Color
Earth	Nose	Nose	Gold
Water	Nose	Mouth	Green
Fire	Mouth	Nose	Red
Air	Mouth	Mouth	Blue

Body Part by Part

Allow about 10–15 minutes for this relaxation exercise. Read very slowly, leaving plenty of time between each instruction. This exercise may be done in a sitting position, legs uncrossed, hands resting on the legs, body tall. When possible, it is preferable to do it lying on the back, legs uncrossed and straight out from the hips, arms at the sides.

Close your eyes, take a few slow and deep breaths, then breathe naturally, preferably through your nose. Allow the mouth to remain slightly open so that you don't clench your teeth or jaw.

If you are lying on your back, let your head roll gently from side to side to be sure there is no tension in your neck, and then bring your head back to center. Each time you inhale, focus on a body part. Each time you exhale, feel that body part softening, relaxing, melting, and letting go.

Starting at the top of your head, concentrate on your scalp as you inhale and, as you exhale, *let go,* feeling every follicle of hair melting away. As you breathe in, pay attention to your forehead; as you exhale, *let go.*

Now bring your attention to your eyebrows, eyelids, and eyes. As you exhale, relax, let go. Bring your consciousness to your ears and your cheeks. As you breathe out, let go. Now focus on your mouth, your teeth and gums, and tongue. When you exhale, feel them melting away.

Imagine two lines beginning at the point of your hairline directly above the bridge of your nose, one going in each direction, following the hairline all the way around your ears and to the nape of your neck, where they meet and then separate again. Continue to imagine these lines traveling around the front to your chin, where they meet before entering your mouth. Now imagine this line traveling around the inside and outside of your lower and upper gums.

Move your attention down to your neck and shoulders, and, as you breathe out, soften, let go, relax. Now let your attention travel down your arms, upper and lower, and relax. Let your mind's eye travel down to your wrists and hands and each and every finger, one at a time. Concentrate on relaxing your right hand—little finger ... ring finger ... middle finger ... index finger ... thumb. Then concentrate on relaxing your left hand—thumb ... index finger ... middle finger ... ring finger ... little finger.

Gently bring your focus to your spine, and allow your mind's eye to travel down your spine, vertebra by vertebra, all the way down to your coccyx bone, the tail end of your spine.

Let your focus travel to your chest and rib cage, feeling the body soften and let go. Place your attention next on your pelvis ... hips ... stomach and buttocks and, as you exhale, relax— relax. Allow your focus to travel down your legs: thighs ... knees and lower legs ... let go. Picture your ankles and feet—letting go of your heels, metatarsals (arches), and the balls of your feet, and one toe at a time, let go. Left foot: big toe ... next toe ... middle toe ... next toe ... little toe. Repeat with the right foot. Feel the weight of your body and the impression it is making on the chair, floor, or bed.

Scan your body, up and down. If you find any places where there is tension, focus your mind on that spot and breathe into it, imagining that spot filling with bubbles of air or white light and, as you exhale, feel the tension float away.

Words to focus on while relaxing besides the words *relax, melt,* and *let go* are: soften, cushion, mellow, yield, give in, liquid like warm oil, soft as butter, like a down quilt, silk, release, free, relinquish, rest, loosen, ease, thaw, and dissolve. Complete the exercise by using some form of reentry.

IMAGERY

Your imagination can take you anywhere you would like to go. You can journey outward as far as you would like in time and space, or inward to the core of your being. You can use imagery as a way to take mini-vacations. There are no limits to what you can imagine. In addition, such visualization has been used very successfully with cancer patients (see Siegel, 1986;

Simonton, Simonton, & Creighton, 1978). Imagery is also an important aspect of stress management training for people with a variety of illnesses and with chronic pain; it is used in such a program at the Harvard Medical School's Body/Mind Institute. The following are some suggested ways of facilitating guided imagery.[1]

Before beginning, you may want to ask the class members to close their eyes and picture their living quarters. Ask them to count the windows, or to see in their minds' eye a favorite painting, photo, or memento in their home. Some people may need a few practice sessions before they are able to envision images. Not everyone sees mental images, but everyone can tell you how many windows he or she has; imagery may be sensory as well as pictorial.

Awakening the Senses with a Lemon

Ask the group to close their eyes and envision holding a lemon. After they have had the chance to visualize the lemon and sense the feel of it, tell them to imagine cutting the lemon in half. Now tell them to slowly lift one half to their mouths and taste it. Many people will actually salivate and make a face that will indicate their response to the sour taste.

Music as an Image Maker

Choose a piece of music without words, such as a piece of classical music, preferably one that may be unfamiliar so that it does not evoke particular memories or images. I like to use music that sounds like outer space, such as "The Music of Cosmos" or Holst's "The Planets" electronically performed by Isko Tomita.

Have the group close their eyes and tell them to let their minds wander freely. Ask them to see what images come to

---

[1]For further information on this subject, see *Creative Visualization* (Gawain, 1989); *Visualization Directing* (Bry, 1979); *Go See the Movie in Your Head* (Shorr, 1977); *Getting Well Again* (Simonton, Simonton, & Creighton, 1978); *Love, Medicine, and Miracles* (Siegel, 1986); and *Guided Imagery* (Moen, 1992). Another book I like to use is *Meditating with Children: The Art of Concentration and Centering* (Rozman, 1975). Although the book is intended for use with children, with some variations I find it applicable for all ages.

them. What pictures does the music evoke? What does it make them think of? Let the music play for 3–5 minutes, giving the group some time to conjure up visions and stories. Bring the group back by slowly turning down the sound of the music and gently asking them to open their eyes. Ask them one at a time to share what they saw.

Freedom Dance

Choose a piece of music without words, preferably an active piece of music, such as Paul Horn's *Inside II* or Jean Michel Jarré's *Equinoxe.* Tell the group to close their eyes and, while continuing to sit, to imagine themselves dancing wherever they want. Tell the group, "You are able to do anything you want, there are no limitations. You can see yourself dancing on a beach, in a meadow, or in a large ballroom—in fact, anywhere because it is your choice; let yourself go."

Let the music play for about 5 minutes and then slowly turn down the sound and ask the group to open their eyes. Start the music over from the beginning and ask the group to stand up and dance as they did in their minds' eyes. Those persons who can't stand or who are shaky on their feet can dance with their arms, heads, torsos, and legs while sitting in their chairs.

Let the music play for about 5 more minutes and then have everyone sit down and share experiences. Some people have imagined themselves in outer space or underwater, and have recounted how the feeling of floating provided them a greater sense of freedom. In my experience, *imagining* dancing or moving with greater freedom often allows people to move with greater range than usual.

Going Places

In this imagery exercise, the facilitator can take the group on an imaginary trip to a place of his or her choice, such as a beach, a forest, or a paradise island. My choice is the beach, and I use a tape of ocean sounds to accompany the exercise.

I begin by asking the group to close their eyes and, after taking a few deep breaths, to relax. Sometimes I lead the group through one of the relaxation exercises described on pages 97–101. Then I ask them to tune into all of their senses and to imagine themselves on a beach.

To facilitate this exercise, read or audiotape the following instructions. Remember to speak slowly, softly, and gently, and to pause for 10–20 seconds after each instruction.

> Hear the sound of the ocean and smell the salt air. See the sun in a fair blue sky. Feel the warmth of the sun on your body. See and feel yourself lying on the beach; feel the impression your body is making in the sand; feel the weight of your body in the sand. You may want to imagine a blanket under your body if the image of lying on the sand is upsetting to you. You may even hear a few seagulls. Envision the edge of the ocean, see the little wave that trickles onto the beach, which glistens like gems in the sun.
>
> Slowly allow yourself to be carried out into a calm sea, smelling the salt air even more strongly because you are so close to it, almost tasting it. As your body floats, feel the coolness of the water under you and the warmth of the sun above you, feeling the coolness even more as the water splashes on the front of your body every now and then. Feel the undulation of the water under you as you continue to float, being aware of the difference that your body feels between floating and the weightedness of lying in the sand.
>
> Now let your mind's eye go to the sky and pick out one puffy cloud in a relatively clear blue sky. This will be your companion cloud. Allow your body to slowly float up next to this cloud and feel the freedom of floating in the air. Feel the breezes and be aware of the different feeling between floating in the air and floating on the water.

Slowly bring the group back to the reality of the moment and ask if anyone would like to share what he or she felt during or after the imagery. This visualization can be followed by a drawing session, letting everyone draw the images they saw.

Your Own Place

After leading the group through one of the relaxation exercises, tell them at the count of three to picture themselves in their favorite place of relaxation, either a place they have been to before, indoors or out, or a place they can make up in their own minds. Tell them that, when they get to this place, they should tune into all their senses: seeing, hearing, smelling, and feeling everything in their chosen surroundings.

If it's indoors, ask them to be aware of what colors are there, where the furniture is, what is on the walls, and what the sounds and smells are. Ask: "Is what you are sitting or standing on soft or hard? Are you alone?" If they are outdoors, ask them to go through the same process with their senses. Then count to three and snap your fingers, saying: "You are now there. See, hear, smell, feel, and taste, if that applies." Tell the group to take about 30 seconds to get accustomed to this place.

Ask them to choose a word, such as *love, peace, calm, clarity*, or any other word they would like. Tell them: "When you have your word, feel this word and its meaning throughout your whole body, in every pore of your being. You now are this word. If your word is *love*, you are love. Love radiates from you and anyone who comes near you becomes love with you." Remind the group, "This word is yours and you can call on it anytime you'd like. You just have to close your eyes, take a few slow deep breaths, count to three, and the feeling is yours again. You own it."

Slowly bring the group back to reality and allow time for sharing and discussion.

Inner Guide

Ask the group to close their eyes and take a few slow and deep breaths, relaxing and letting go of their bodies and minds. Then tell them they are going on a journey. Each person should think of a question he or she wants answered, or a problem he or she needs help with. To facilitate this exercise, read or audiotape the following instructions, speaking slowly, softly, and gently. Pause long enough to give everyone the chance to experience each of the suggested activities, and allow a minute or more for each to start a conversation with his or her inner guide.

> Imagine that your are going through a door opening out to a path that goes up a mountain on a beautiful spring day. Feel the breezes and smell the fresh mountain air. As you walk, you will pass lovely trees and plants, some with fragrant scents. You may even decide to pause and bend down to smell or pick a flower or two. As you continue up this path, you may see squirrels, rabbits, or other playful creatures of nature. A little further up the mountain, you will come to a bubbling brook and you may want to stop to take a drink, or run your finger through the water. You may even decide to rest, to take off your shoes and dangle your feet in the water.
>
> At your own pace, you may continue when you please on your way up the path. Further along the path, you will encounter

your guide. This guide may be in any shape or form, human or otherwise. When you do meet your guide, start a conversation. Get to know your guide and then ask your question. When you have concluded your encounter, say your farewells. Know that you can meet again whenever you choose, and slowly retrace your steps to return down the path and back through the door.

Give everyone a few minutes and then remind them that, if they haven't already started their journeys back, it is now time to do so. You may want to lead them back, or you can allow them to return on their own.

Afterward, it is a good idea to have a sharing discussion when the group is ready. There may be some people who did not meet their guide. Assure them that it sometimes happens that way, and that perhaps next time they will. Whether or not they did so, if they did not get an answer to their question, it may come to them at another time, perhaps when they least expect it.

Alice in Wonderland

This is a visualization that can help place a specific relationship into a different perspective. Have each person think of a close relationship they have with someone, such as a mate; a child; a close friend; or, if in a long-term care facility, a nurse or caregiver. Then ask everyone to close his or her eyes, take a few slow and deep breaths, and let go, relaxing body and mind.

Lead into this imagery by saying:

Imagine yourself with this person you have chosen, and picture where you are, indoors or outdoors. If indoors, which room are you sitting in? Is it at a table, or on a sofa, or other setting? If outdoors, are you on a patio, a lawn, a beach? Where are you sitting? When you have decided where you are, see yourself and your partner in this place, and start an imaginary conversation.

Give the group a few moments for each person to establish this conversation in his or her mind and then continue:

You will notice that a bottle will appear in your right hand. On this bottle is a tag that will say, "Drink me" and, like Alice in Wonderland, you will drink the contents of the bottle, and you will begin to become very small, as small as Tom Thumb, as small as a thimble. But you will continue your conversation with this person, whose size does not change, noticing how you feel physically and emotionally. How does it feel to be so small, so tiny? How does your body feel? How do you feel in the environment; in the furniture? Does your conversation change? How is your partner treating you, and how are you relating to and responding to this person?

Allow a few moments for this scenario to develop. Then continue.

Now you will notice that a bottle has appeared in your left hand. A tag on this bottle reads, "Drink me." You drink the contents of this bottle and, like Alice in Wonderland, you find yourself growing larger and larger until you are giant size, filling the entire room you are in, with your head touching the ceiling, unless you are outside. Your partner, meanwhile, has remained the same size, and your conversation has continued. Again, be aware of how you feel being so large, towering over the person you are with. How does your body feel; your clothes; the furniture? How do you feel emotionally? Has your conversation changed? How are you relating now? How is this person treating you, and how are you treating this person?

Allow a few moments of this scenario to be established and then continue.

At this point another bottle will appear in your hand, and it too will have a tag on it that says, "Drink me." You will drink the contents of this bottle and then find yourself shrinking back to your normal size. Your partner and you will continue to talk while this is happening and, when you reach your normal size, you will find a way to complete your conversation. Slowly open your eyes and return to the group.

Follow this exercise with a sharing discussion. Ask what each person learned about him- or herself and their relationship with the person they had chosen. Ask, "When you became small, did you feel vulnerable or frightened, or were you carefree and playful? Did the person you were with take care of you, baby you, protect you, or take advantage of you and bully you or patronize you? When you became enormous, did your partner cower, or treat you with more respect?" Use the discussion time to recognize, vent, and share feelings.

THE IMPORTANCE OF TOUCH

"The raw sensation of stimulus is vitally necessary for the physical survival of the organism.... The basic need for tactile stimulation must be added to the repertoire of basic needs in all vertebrates" (Montague, 1971, p. 332). Touching, in our culture, is intimidating to some; yet it is very important. The skin is the largest sense organ we have and is involved with everything "that goes on outside the organism" (Montague, 1971, p. 2). The opportunity to touch and be touched is often lacking in the lives of older adults. Some may no longer have a spouse, and many have minimal or no contact with young children, who are wonderful about unself-consciously climbing on your lap and putting their arms around you. Touch is particularly important to persons with cognitive impairment, who may repeatedly stroke or pat things or who have busy hands that just can't stay still. These individuals enjoy touch as an activity with objects and enjoy being a receiver of caring touch.

There is a natural healing power in the exchange and the warmth of touch. According to Goleman (1988), it was theorized by Dr. Seymour Levine from Stanford University Medical School that, in humans, a touch-induced reduction of stress hormones may account for the soothing effects of skin-to-skin contact. In his book, *Living, Loving & Learning,* Leo Buscaglia quotes Dr. Harold Falk, senior psychiatrist at the Menninger Foundation: "Hugging can lift depression, enabling the body's immunization system to become tuned up. Hugging breathes fresh life into tired bodies and makes you feel younger and more vibrant. In the home, hugging can strengthen relationships and significantly reduce tensions" (1982, p. 237). Buscaglia further states,

> Helen Colton in her book, *Joy of Touching,* said that the hemoglobin is that part of the blood that carries the vital supplies of oxygen to the heart and to the brain—and she says that if you want to be healthy, you must touch each other, you must love each other, you must hold each other. (p. 237)

After a class has been meeting for awhile and I feel confident that they would be comfortable with touch, I introduce some tactile experiences. I end all my classes with shared hugs (Figure 29), sometimes waiting until after a few initial meetings with a new class. Therefore, by the time I present touch-related activities, everyone has already touched. It is important from the beginning to establish a safe environment where the participants feel secure in the fact that they have permission to

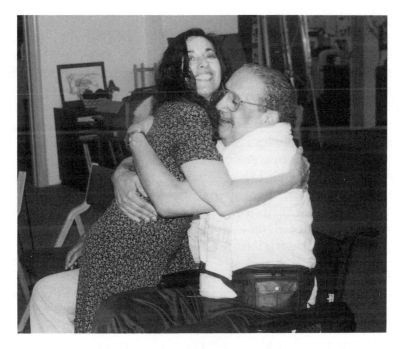

Figure 29.   Hugging fills the need for tactile stimulation.

be comfortable with themselves and the group. It is a good idea to preface these activities by mentioning that those who wish not to take part need not do so. Those with arthritis may not be able to tolerate touch. Because very frail persons are not mobile enough to participate, I sometimes go to each and give the opportunity to experience touching. I have found these touch-related activities to be among the favorites in every group, and they are often requested. Many people are amazed by the warmth they can feel from the hands, and often feel better afterward.

After any touch-related activity, remind the group that it is a good idea to wash their hands after the session. This is a particularly good idea in case the session takes place before a meal.

Hands-On

Tell the members of the group to find a partner and move their chairs so that they are facing each other. Then give them the following instructions:

- Close your eyes, place your own hands together, and rub them. As you breathe deeply, mentally focus your breath into your hands.
- Now, with eyes open, place your hands (palms touching, fingers and thumbs up) on your partner's hands. Once again close your eyes. Breathe deeply and focus your mind on the hands. Feel the warmth. Very slowly lessen the pressure so that you are barely touching, yet continue to feel the warmth.
- Now, with eyes open or closed, move your hands a fraction of an inch away and then touch again. Continue to do this and move further and further, going forward and touching and then away again, to and fro, like a magnet. See how far you can go and still feel the heat of your partner's hands. (See "Hand Dances with Partners" in Chapter 4.)

Shoulder Massage

Tell the group to partner up. Have one partner sit and the other stand behind the partner's chair. The person sitting should close his or her eyes and take a few deep breaths to relax. The person standing should place his or her hands together as in the previous activity. (I tell my classes that before placing my hands on someone, I like to close my eyes and ask to be a channel for a higher source. Then I let them decide what feels right for them.) Then give the standing partners the following instructions:

- After you have taken a few deep breaths, place your hands gently on top of your partner's shoulders (Figure 30), close to the neck, with your fingers in the front and the palms and heels of the hand toward the back. Just let the warmth of your hands feel the warmth of your partner's shoulders while you both focus on this area and do some deep relaxed breathing.
- Now gently squeeze your hands, squeezing the shoulder area. Slowly continue this movement while you move your hands outward toward the edge of the shoulder and back again toward the neck. (The sitting partner is free to express preference for a firmer or gentler touch.)
- Next, make circles with the thumb (be sure to use the padded part and not the nail), gently massaging the shoulder area along muscle and not bone. Finish with still and quiet hands, as when you started.

- Both of you should take a few deep breaths. Then brush your hands gently outward along your partner's shoulders, just like you were brushing off some lint. End by shaking out your hands.

At the end of the exercise, the partners can change places and repeat the whole process.

This activity can be extended by having the seated person bend his or her torso forward so that the partner can reach the shoulder blades and more of the spine. Tell the massaging partners that they can gently run their fingers along the inside of the shoulder blades next to the spine, just off the bone where all the muscles are attached.

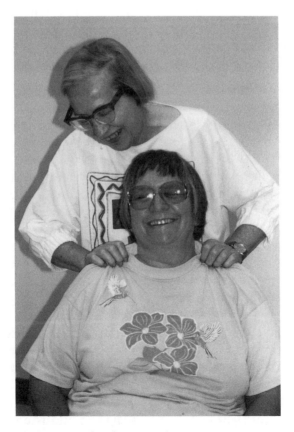

Figure 30.   A hands-on exercise.

Hand Massage

Tell the group to pick partners. Have both partners sit in chairs and take turns gently massaging each other's hands according to the following instructions:

- Take the time to do each and every finger. Place your first finger and thumb on the top and bottom of each knuckle, making circles working down to the fingertip. Then place a finger and a thumb on the sides of each finger, making circles working down to the fingertip.
- Now try stretching the fingers back gently, then pulling each finger gently.
- Be sure to massage the palms and the top of the hands between the bones.
- Finish by gently stretching each hand from the wrist, up and down, as if you were waving hello. Now, without forcing, circle the hand from the wrist in both directions. Then hold the hand between your two hands, again focusing on breath and warmth.

Tell the group that, if they feel their own hands need circulation or they have some pain in the hands, they do not need a partner; they can do this activity at any time for themselves.

Polarity

Another touch-related activity uses the warmth of the hands at different places on the body at the same time. This can be done on one's own body, or with a partner. Tell the group to place a part of the body that is tense or in pain in between their right and left hands. An example would be to place the right hand on the front of a knee and the left hand on back of the knee.

You can have the class experiment by each taking a partner and practicing on an arm, leg, shoulder, or even the head. (This can also be done by participants themselves, without a partner.) Have the touching partners rub their palms together to cause friction and warmth, as in the Hands-On activity. After placing the hands in a polarity position (one front and one back on a knee, or one top and one bottom on an arm, or on either side, as at the temples of a head), ask the group to close their eyes and focus on their breathing and the connection between the hands. This often is felt as a healing energy. Be sure everyone has a turn at being both the touching partner and the receiving partner.

Chapter 9

Awakening Awareness

We believe life should be added to years as well as years added to life.

—Sister Pat Murphy, *Aging & Spirituality*

Most of us walk around with our senses and perceptions dulled. Some of us purposely shield ourselves from the sights and sounds we prefer not seeing and hearing and get into habits of being single focused and tunnel visioned.

Our awareness can be stretched and expanded at any age. Once we are nudged awake and given reminders and tools to open our perceptions, it is as if a window has been opened and we can see and hear outside of the little rooms that are ourselves, into the environment around us.

PERCEPTION EXPANDERS

Five ideas to help expand perception are suggested below. These activities are not appropriate for participants who are confused, or who have visual impairment.

Learning to Look and See

Have everyone look around the room for 1 minute. Then tell them to close their eyes and ask them questions, such as, "What color is the floor? What color is the ceiling? Are there pictures on the walls? Can you describe the walls and what's on them? Are there windows? Can you describe the window coverings and the furniture? What is the person on your right wearing? What am I wearing?" More open-ended questions, such as "What did you see?" can also be used. Encourage detailed descriptions.

Taking an Observational Walk

If possible, have the group take a 10- to 15-minute walk somewhere in the building or outside. Discuss everyone's observations when you return. I have had groups come back from observational walks on which one person noticed the wiring that went all around a wall, another noticed colors, another heard bits and pieces of conversations, and another noticed what people were wearing or how animated their conversations were. Some people are aware of visual details (e.g., the wiring), some are more observant of what they hear, others notice colors, and yet others focus their attention on people and their gestures.

Noticing Details About Your Partner

Have each participant face a partner and observe him or her, taking note of as many details as possible in a few minutes. Then tell the participants to turn their chairs away from each other and change 3–10 things about themselves (e.g., remove some jewelry, move a ring or bracelet from one hand to another, take off one shoe, roll up a sleeve). After a given amount of time, have them turn back to their partners and see how many changed items each can detect.

Perceiving Change

Before the group enters the room, change something about the room and see who notices and how long it takes before someone notices the change. Wear something obviously different once in a while and see if anyone notices.

Drawing a Path

Have each person draw a simple shape, such as a letter of the alphabet or a simple geometric shape. Then have everyone, one at a time, either walk out the shape in a path on the floor or draw the shape in the air with a body part. Have them repeat this twice and ask them to say when they are beginning and when they are done. Next, on another piece of paper, have everyone else draw the shape they perceived, and then share the shapes to see how many variations there are.

After the group has seen all the shapes, ask them to choose a mixture of four or five shapes that includes curved lines, straight lines, and zigzag lines, as seen in a triangle, the letter S, and the letter M. The four or five people chosen should move simultaneously, each starting at a different point in the center of the circle and going in a different direction. This can be developed into a dance by changing the walks to runs and skips and changing their level and direction. Add music or rhythmic accompaniment and repetitions of each person's moving shape. It is fun to choose a partner for each person and have that partner accompany the moving person with a sound or musical instrument. This activity encourages everyone to watch carefully, to pay close attention to what they see, and then to reproduce what they have seen.

SENSES

Information comes to us through our senses. The keener our awareness and perception, the greater our learning skills. The more conscious we are of our senses, the easier it is to make the connection to our cognitive selves.

As we mature, the senses often diminish. Therefore, using our senses more frequently with a conscious focus on each sense is important. Enhancing observational skills is significant for anyone, and particularly for people with special needs. We often are so concerned with people's disabilities, that we forget about something as basic as awareness of senses. Fully exploring each sense offers the opportunity for a richer experience of life.

"Don't forget to stop and smell the roses" is a cliché we often hear. In a workshop I once took with Brian Way, a British expert on creative dramatics, he noted:

> Just think what would happen if we didn't comb our hair, brush our teeth, or bathe for 3 days? Yet how many of us spend just 5 minutes a day focusing on our senses—to stop and see as we look, to explore with our eyes in detail, to stop and hear as we

listen—tuning in to all the sounds. How often do we actually feel what we touch and allow ourselves the pleasure of examining and perhaps seeing with our hands and fingers; to slow down and taste what we eat and to remember to smell the flowers as well as the scents of all things as we move through our day?

It's true that we often put up screens to protect ourselves from the unpleasant and the bombardment of our senses. But along the way, many of us have deadened our senses so that we have lost an important part of our sense of self.

Touch

One of the methods I use to enhance the sense of touch is to explore different textures, such as feathers (Figure 31), sandpaper, tape, rubber bands, and cold cream. Before presenting these textures, I ask participants to touch and notice the feel of their clothes, shoes, skin, hair, fingernails, the chair they are sitting in, and the floor. When possible, I ask them to walk around the room while noticing the feel of things in and around the room. While they are experiencing by touching, I ask them to think about whether what they are touching is rough, smooth, bumpy, cold, warm, sticky, and so forth.

A short discussion follows this initial touch experience. Often there are people who are surprised by the feel of things

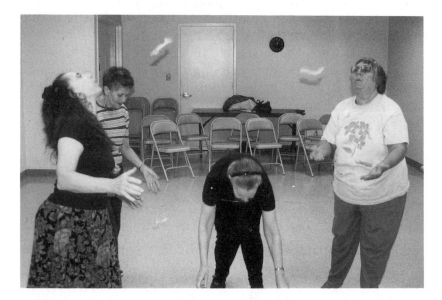

Figure 31.   Moving with feathers to explore their qualities.

they see every day but don't normally pay attention to. Then we proceed with the exploration of the above-listed textures, one at a time. After exploring each texture, we discuss the qualities of each, and what each is like. For example, I ask, "What does the feather feel like?" Some of the responses are: "A feather is soft, light, and tickly," and "It floats and twirls when you blow on it." I ask the participants to mention something else that feels like a feather. Some responses are: "It is like snow." "It is like birds." "It is like a pillow." This discussion is followed by movement, first with a body part and then with the whole body, that represents the quality and properties of each texture. Suitable music is chosen for each texture to help motivate movement. (I use "Ave Maria" for the feathers.) This activity allows the participants to have fun while moving and thinking.

With some groups it is difficult to get responses. The group facilitator may need to make some of the following suggestions for the qualities and properties of the remaining textures:

- *Sandpaper* is rough, sandy, and jerky. It is like a stubble beard, toast, cement, an emery board, or a nail file. Representative movement would be jerky, and probably quick. The music I use for this texture is "Flight of the Bumble Bee," by Rimsky-Korsakov.
- *Rubber bands* are smooth and rubbery. They shake like Jell-O, stretch like elastic or chewing gum, wiggle like a worm, snap across the room, and make shapes. Representative movement would be wiggling, making shapes, and stretching slowly and quickly. The music I use for this texture is "Finlandia," by Sibelius.
- *Tape* is like glue, paste, wet cement, Velcro, and taffy. Representative movement would be quick and jerky, or like pulling metal away from a strong magnet. For this texture, I use African music from Ghana.
- *Cold cream* is smooth, cool, creamy, slimy, sensual, silky, and slippery. It is like body oil, butter, and mayonnaise. Representative movement might be slithering, sliding, and melting. The music I use for this texture is "Clair de Lune," by Debussy.

With participants with visual impairments, it is a good idea to have them sit next to you—or, if you are fortunate enough to have an aide, to have them sit next to the aide. Usually anyone sitting next to this person who is capable of doing so—participant, observer, or assistant—is glad to be of assistance.

Textures can be collected on a nature walk or brought in from home. If one texture is presented at each session, it may be possible to include drawings that depict the quality of the texture or the texture itself. The participants can also express their feelings and memories about the texture in a word or sentence that could be developed in a poem or story.

I have found that textures can awaken and motivate people when nothing else can. In one nursing home, a woman who had just lost her vision responded only minimally to most of what I did. When we worked with texture, however, she became totally involved. After each person had had the chance to feel and experience each of the texture samples I had passed out, I collected them. The blind woman did not want to relinquish her sandpaper. I told her that if she was to keep the sandpaper, she'd have to have a feather in her other pocket for balance and gave them both to her. After that, she took part in more of the activities that we did.

Slowing down, sensing the object you are feeling, can be a spiritual experience. Truly sensing is being totally with—perhaps becoming one with—that which we are sensing.

Hearing and Listening

To enhance the sense of hearing and the pleasure of listening, try the following activities:

- Tell the participants to close their eyes and listen to the sounds around them, inside and outside. After a minute or two of silence, have them share what they heard with the group.
- Play a piece of music and let everyone share the images that come to mind after a few minutes.
- Add drawing to either of the previous activities.

Smell

To enhance the sense of smell, bring in envelopes and blotters with various scents in or on them (e.g., cinnamon, oregano, mint, tea, coffee, and pepper in envelopes; ammonia, rose oil, coconut oil, and alcohol on blotters). Discuss memories of some of the scents. A memory can be expressed in an oral history, poem, drawing, creative movement, or mime, and expanded into a dance. Music and sound effects could be added to enhance the dramatic effect.

Taste

To enhance the sense of taste, cut out pictures of food and discuss the taste of each, as well as some of the memories connected with them. Bring in various foods and conduct a taste test, with blindfolded participants either guessing the food or describing the taste of each food. (Be certain ahead of time that there are no allergies or health or religious restrictions on any of the foods you are using.)

A Multisensory Exercise with Peanuts

In this activity, the group explores a peanut with each of the five senses. First, each participant takes a peanut in the shell from a bag that is passed around. Examining the peanut carefully for a few minutes will acquaint each person with the specific aspects of his or her "personal" peanut. The group can then be paired off, with each pair putting its peanuts together, mixing them up to see if each person can identify his or her original peanut (Figure 32). This process is repeated with three or four people in a group and then with larger numbers of people. In my experience, individuals are able to find their own peanut with no difficulty most of the time.

The second part of this process has the participants examine their peanuts with their eyes closed, touching and feeling each crevice, crack, and bump of the peanut. Then, the above process of pairing off into partners, followed by threesomes and then larger groups, is repeated, with all participants closing their eyes and finding their own peanuts by sense of touch.

Next, with eyes open, have the participants smell the peanut while it is still in its shell. Ask them to place it next to their ears and crack it open. The sound of the cracking shell is magnified and very different when it is right next to the ear. (Of course, this may not work for people with diminished hearing or a hearing impairment.)

Continue to explore slowly the inside of the shell and the peanut by touch and smell. The inner shell is very smooth and

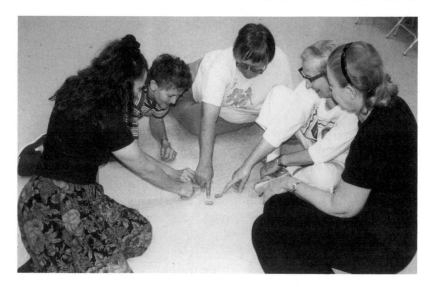

Figure 32.   Participants point to their own peanuts.

silky and the scent becomes stronger. Participants should notice the color and feel of the peanut skin, and listen to it as they remove it very slowly, perhaps smelling it and then tasting it. The skin may seem papery and bitter. Before the participants actually place the peanut in their mouths, have them feel its smoothness. Tell them to part it in half, noting the little knob inside at the top, and smelling it again. (Before the tasting part of this activity, ask if there are any dietary restrictions or dental problems with peanuts.)

When they place the peanut in their mouth, they may want to roll it around the tongue and under, feeling it against the inside of the cheeks and the roof of the mouth as well as the gums. When they do bite into it, ask them to do so very slowly, feeling and tasting the juice. Encourage them to continue to bite into the peanut slowly so that they can feel the texture changing from peanut to peanut butter, crunchy to smooth, as well as the stronger taste of the peanut.

After the exercise is over, hold a discussion with the group in which you talk about the stronger awareness of each of the senses stimulated by this process before proceeding with the imagery exercise.

When the discussion is over, ask the group to close their eyes and imagine themselves as peanuts inside shells (Figure

33). What does it feel like being this size and shape? What does it smell like? Is it dark or light? Do you feel safe? confined? neither? What can you hear? How can you move?

For participants who cannot stand, the following activity can be done with a single body part. Those who can stand may want to hold onto the backs of their chairs; those who are able to can get down on the floor. Ask the group to imagine themselves in a bowl with other peanuts. Ask them to move accordingly, imagining that the bowl is being passed around and shaken, then emptied into a pan and the peanuts roasted. Imagine that some of the peanuts are dumped out of the bowl and roll away.

After this imagery, the group can share experiences and discuss the feelings and thoughts that may have emerged during the exercise.

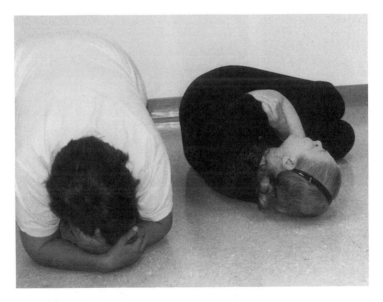

Figure 33.   Pretending to be peanuts inside a shell.

Chapter 10

Reminiscing
and Motivating
Communication

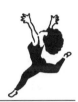

Youth is happy because it has the ability to see beauty.
Anyone who keeps the ability to see beauty never grows old.
—Franz Kafka

For those who have not worked with many older adults, it is important to become aware of and overcome stereotyped perceptions[1]. Many older adults themselves have been conditioned to expect and accept memory loss by biased and ageist negative views ingrained in our culture. The following activities help to trigger old memories and serve to remind older adults that they have lived rich and valuable lives and still have much to share.

REMEMBERING AND SHARING

Simple conversations can be used to activate memories and encourage sharing. Comparisons between past and present can be made to feed the conversations. Sometimes common experiences are discovered among group members: even if this is not the case, discussing such experiences always brings the group closer together because they have shared personal stories and learned more about each other. These exchanges are stimu-

---

[1] I highly recommend *Truth About Aging: Guidelines for Accurate Communications* (American Association of Retired Persons, 1984) as a source for unbiased information about older adults.

lating and help the group become more socially interactive. When the buzz of verbal interaction occurs, thereby increasing the energy level, it is easier to get people moving and there is more physical interaction. When sharing, the participants become more animated and excited, which in itself is physical action.

Sometimes group sharing develops out of my sharing something that has happened to me. My favorite story to share is what happened at one of my birthday celebration parties. Russ T., one of my three sons, arrived from out of town the evening before the party with two of his friends, whom I know well because they had all grown up together. They brought an enormous box into my apartment and said it was a surprise present that I couldn't open until right before the party. They warned me that I wasn't to go near it, touch it, or smell it.

All the next day we decorated the apartment and prepared food for the party. Whenever I happened to be near the box, they would scream at me to get away from it. Just before I went to get dressed for the party, my younger son, Kevin, called from out of town to wish me a happy birthday and to tell me that he was sorry he couldn't be with me but was there in spirit. Feeling touched and happy, I went to get dressed. When I came back into the living area, I was told by Russ T. that I could now open my gift. I slowly began opening the box, and suddenly out jumped my younger son. It was the biggest surprise I had ever received in my life. I was so shocked that my mind was in a state of confusion. I could not think; my mind ran on: "Was he in the box all night?" "How did he call me from the box?" As it turned out, Kevin had just come in by train, called me from one block away, and had been sneaked into the apartment and into the box while I dressed. After sharing this story with the group, I ask for other surprise stories.

There are many other topics I use to stimulate conversation, including your earliest memory of your birthday; your favorite birthday; your first day at school; your earliest Christmas memory; your favorite Christmas or other special holiday; your first boyfriend/girlfriend; things you have done with your hands, legs, body, or life; and what you remember most about the town where you grew up. For example, when asked if she remembered her first boyfriend, one woman answered, "Remember him? I married him!" A group at the Cole Senior Center mentioned the following activities in a discussion of things they had done with their hands:

"Hoed and picked cotton."

"Drew water out of the well."

"Made white lightning. Had a still and used the corn whiskey for medicinal purposes."

"Culled hops. I would place it in a jar and put rock candy in it, let it soak and it would get syrupy. When diluted, it would break up asthma spells for children."

On special holidays, such as Thanksgiving, Mother's Day, and, depending on the ethnic background of the group, Passover or Martin Luther King Day, I have discussions about past experiences with these holidays and ask how each person plans to celebrate the holiday. Sometimes we put these memories together into a poem (see Chapter 12). I have heard some wonderful stories. For example, on one Martin Luther King Day, Helen Maul, an African American woman from the Cole Senior Center, recalled the 1968 riots in Washington, D.C., when all schools and government buildings were closed and government workers were released from work early.

> It was the first time in my 20 years of work at the Commerce Department building that I had seen the iron doors shut. While we were waiting for our husbands to come pick us up, one white woman was hysterical because her husband had called to say he couldn't get across the bridge into D.C. She asked several people if she could get a ride to Southeast, where her husband could pick her up. We had heard that several white persons had been injured with rocks thrown by angry young blacks into their cars. One man and his wife agreed to take her if she was willing to lie on the floor in the back. On our way home, my husband and I ran into a detour where rioting was going on. We had to go out to the Maryland line. Young blacks lined the streets and stoned all cars with whites in them, breaking windshields and windows. Cars with blacks were told to go through. Maryland state troopers with machine guns were daring the young blacks to come over the line with their rocks.

This was an intense moment in our history, and Helen Maul was there in the midst of it. There are so many stories older adults have to tell—a wealth of rich and funny stories; a lifetime of stories for us to learn from and for them to share.

I also use songs as topics for discussion and dance. I play the tape of "Grandma's Hands," a song by Bill Withers, and then ask each person for a hand movement that we then put into a hand dance to the song, or I ask what each person remembers about his or her grandmother or grandfather. One woman got teary eyed reminiscing about how she loved to take walks with her grandfather. In sharing that story, she was also sharing her feelings. Often, older people with cognitive impairment speak of their parents or even grandparents as if they were still alive. These expressed emotions will be very real to them, and should be affirmed. As Naomi Feil advises in *The Validation Breakthrough* (1993), facilitators should avoid contradicting, arguing, or using logic with disoriented people, responding instead to their emotional needs. You might respond by saying, "You must love your grandparents very much."

Another song I play is "My Favorite Things" from *The Sound of Music.* Then each person shares a favorite thing of theirs, which we make into a mime dance. While playing the spiritual, "Lay Your Burden Down," I ask the group to metaphorically find ways to place each of their burdens down, finding different ways to place things of different sizes and weights down on the floor. After this song, I like to ask everyone to say what they are thankful for. (I also ask this question at Thanksgiving.) I have gotten a wonderful variety of responses, ranging from the humorous to the serious to the very basic, such as food and shelter.

"Best You Can Do" and "You're A Friend of Mine" by Bill Withers are both upbeat songs. I ask people to develop a personalized dance to them. Then I ask each person to go into the center of our circle and do his or her dance one at a time while the rest follow. After everyone has had a turn in the center, we all go back to doing our own dance. With very frail elderly persons, I hold their hands and dance with them one at a time. I ask the rest to keep the beat by clapping and dancing with as many body parts as they like.

"When The Saints Go Marching In" is a great picker-upper. You can make up words about moving the body and body parts:

> When the saints go marching in,
> When the saints go marching in,
> Oh, I want to be in that number,
> When the saints go marching in!

(Clap your hands)
When we all clap our hands,
When we all clap our hands,
Oh, I want to be in that number,
When we all clap our hands!

(Stomp your feet)
When we all stomp our feet,
When we all stomp our feet,
Oh, I want to be in that number,
When we all stomp our feet!

Tell the class to clap their hands over their heads, behind their backs, and any other places they can think of; ask how many different ways they can think of stomping their feet. You may want to give a few suggestions. With each new stanza of this song, the group can add any body movement they would like; for each new stanza, ask a few people, one at a time, to suggest another body movement. You and members of your class can make up your own movement songs to any rhythm, such as:

Put your hands up to the ceiling,
Stomp your feet and clap your hands.

Old children's songs, such as the "Hokey Pokey," are often fun and are appreciated by older adults. Many old dances, such as the "Bunny Hop" and "Alley Cat," are also fun to do.

Any of these communication initiators can be developed into an activity involving other arts. Each person can do a drawing depicting the subject, or a group mural project can be developed. Mime and movement can be created and either put to music or developed into a drama. Old photographs of grandparents or hometowns can be brought in to be made into a collage. New photos can be taken for pictures of "My Favorite Things" or "What I Am Thankful For."

COMMUNICATION MOTIVATORS

Say Something Nice to Each Person in the Group

Have one person in the group sit or stand in the center of the circle and slowly turn to each person in the circle as each expresses something he or she likes or feels about the person in the center. Typical comments are: "I like the way you always have a smile for everyone," "The bright colors you wear cheer me up," "I admire your flexibility," or "I'm glad you are a part of this group." When each member of the group has made a comment, the person in the center can return to the circle and another can go to the center, and so on until everyone has had a chance to receive comments. Be sure to remind everyone to be sincere, and to find something to say that will be honest, even if it is to say, "I don't know you well enough yet to know what I like about you." If that is the case, then you can suggest that they pair up the next time there is an activity that requires partners.

This Is Your Life

Once a month you can feature the life story of one member of your group. You can do this either in an interview format or by simply letting them tell you their life story and audiotaping the whole thing. Some of the questions you can ask are:

"Tell us your earliest memory."
"Describe the town and the house you grew up in; your family when you were a child; and the kinds of activities you did with your family and your friends."
"What were your teenage years like?"
"Tell us about your courtship and your early marriage."
"What about your vacations and trips?"
"How many children and grandchildren do you have?"
"If you had one piece of advice to give to your grandchildren or the children of this generation, what would it be?"

HOMEWORK REMINDERS

As part of each session, I often like to give the class what I call a "thought reminder." I tell them this is their homework for the week or until I see them next. The next time we meet, I might ask for feedback: "Who remembered, and what happened?"

Examples of some thought reminders include:

1. **Watch your thinking** We often bring ourselves down or keep ourselves in a depressed state by focusing on negative thoughts. Be aware of how often you say "Isn't it awful?" or "terrible," or "sad." There are those who can't wait to

tell you a tragic event. I call them "the bad news bearers." It's true life has awful, terrible, and sad events, but there are also beautiful, joyous, and uplifting events. I believe it is important to focus on the positive rather than the negative. And we can do this without burying our heads in the sand. Practice saying, "Isn't it beautiful?", "Isn't it wonderful?", and "Isn't it magic?", and look for those aspects in life.

2. **Be Good to Yourself** Give yourself permission to do something for yourself every day. Make the time to rest if you need to; cook yourself something special; visit with a friend; call someone who's on your mind. Make a list of the things that give you pleasure and pick one each day to do for yourself. (Nursing home residents can visit with a neighbor in another room, make a call to someone special, make up a box of special treats [food, jokes, poems, or old letters], or spray on a favorite scent.)

3. **Find Things to Laugh About** Humor is so important. Don't forget to be able to laugh at yourself. This is a good reminder for us all when we get bogged down or become too intense. Bring in a funny story to share about something that happened to you or something you heard or read about. Set aside a day when each group member relates a humorous anecdote.

    Joel Goodman, director of the Humor Project in Saratoga Springs, New York, suggests making a humor "first-aid kit." Collect all the jokes, funny magazines, videotapes, or whatever tickles your fancy in a special box or drawer.

4. **Be Extra Considerate** Most people are considerate most of the time. Pick one day and be extra conscientious about everyone you come in contact with and extend yourself beyond the norm. Practice random acts of kindness.

5. **Practice Eye Contact** Make eye contact when you communicate with someone, even if your verbal exchange is brief, such as with the checkout counter person at the market. Try to make eye contact with as many people as you can; practice on other members of the class. Say hello to more people, even strangers. You will be amazed how many smiles you collect when you notice and acknowledge someone.

THOUGHT FOR THE DAY

I often bring in quotations for contemplation. These can come from anywhere—poetry, spiritual material, or even something someone I know said. Whenever I come across a good quotation, I file it away. I now have a collection of quotes, thoughts, sayings, and affirmations. These quotations can be used for remembering and sharing or to promote conversation among group members. The group can be encouraged to start their own files of quotations. You could also have a special bulletin board for uplifting "quotes for the day"; group members can bring in quotations they find to post on the board.

After sharing one of my quotations, I might ask if anyone has any comment or response. Sometimes I just give the quote in our closing circle, and say it's the "thought for the day," without any further discussion. The following quotations are some of the ones that I use.

The only gift is a portion of thyself...
—Ralph Waldo Emerson

I believe in the sun even when it is not shining,
I believe in love even when I feel it not,
I believe in God even when He is silent.
—Sign found on a concentration camp wall

(I read this during a workshop I was giving, as an example of some of the "thoughts for the day," and one of the participants shared a story related to this. She said, "When I was in a museum in Israel, sitting with a group of people in a ship that had brought Jews to Israel, someone in the group recited the same quotation from memory. When she finished the quote, a woman in the group named Ruth Kluger said, 'I was the one who wrote that.' " The next time I presented a workshop, at another conference in D.C., I told this story and a minister who was one of the participants in this workshop informed me that music had been written to this and it was in a children's song book. He later mailed me a copy of the music.)

A woman noticed that when her life was going well for her and she took her usual walk on the beach, there were two sets of footprints. But when she was depressed or things were hard for her there was only one set of prints.

*During a bad depression, she spoke to the Lord and
asked, "Why is it when I really need you, you're not there?"
And the Lord answered, "Dearest, the times you have
seen only one set of prints are the times I have carried you!"*
—Unknown

The following is a letter written by Benjamin Franklin to
Miss Hubbard on the occasion of the death of his brother,
John Franklin:

*Philadelphia, 23rd Feb., 1756. I condole with you. We
have lost a most dear and valuable relation. But it is the will
of God and nature that these mortal bodies be laid aside
when the soul is to enter into real life. This is rather an
embryo state, a preparation for living. A man is not
completely born until he be dead. Why, then, should we grieve
that a new child is born among the immortals, a new member
added to their happy society?*

*We are spirits. That bodies should be lent us while they
can afford us pleasure, assist us in acquiring knowledge, or in
doing good to our fellow-creatures, is a kind and benevolent
act of God. When they become unfit for these purposes and
afford us pain instead of pleasure, instead of an aid become
an encumbrance, and answer none of the intentions for which
they were given, it is equally kind and benevolent that a way
is provided by which we may get rid of them. Death is that
way. We ourselves, in some cases, prudently choose a partial
death. A mangled, painful limb which cannot be restored
we willingly cut off. He who plucks out a tooth parts with
it freely, since the pain goes with it; and he who quits the
whole body parts with all pains and possibilities of pains
and diseases which it was liable to or capable of making
him suffer.*

*Our friend and we were invited abroad on a party of
pleasure which is to last forever. We could not all conveniently
start together, and why should you and I be grieved at this,
since we are soon to follow and know where to find him?
Adieu, B. Franklin....*

*There is no such thing as a "bad experience," but only
opportunities to learn and grow in inner understanding....
Our stumbling blocks are stepping stones.*
—Ruth Montgomery, *Strangers Among Us*

He who has a WHY to live can bear with almost any HOW....

[E]verything can be taken from a man but one thing: the last of the human freedoms—to choose one's attitude in any given set of circumstances: to choose one's own way.
                    —Victor E. Frankel, *Man's Search for Meaning*

[You] do have a terminal illness: it's called death. A few years more or less time before you are washed away makes little difference. Be happy now, without reason—or you never will be at all...

Act happy, feel happy, be happy, without a reason in the world. Then you can love, and do what you will.
                    —Dan Millman, *Way of the Peaceful Warrior*

If you are ignorant, old age is a famine. If you are learned it is a harvest....

One becomes what one displays....

When people have made peace with death, they live with greater consciousness. Every day, every moment becomes more complete in itself. It makes people impatient with trivia, decorum, deception, because every moment counts, for good or ill.
                    —Barbara Myerhoff, *Number Our Days*

Each one of us determines the beliefs by which he lives.... Our world is not held together by our worrying about it. We can lead a life that is free of fear. Just as I am, you are the determiner of everything that happens to you....

An attitude can heal...simply think what it pleases you to think, what rests and comforts you...simply take careful notice of what makes you happy to think, and what makes you unhappy, and your mind will make the necessary adjustments itself....

Words are irrelevant to what we teach and learn...The EXPERIENCE of love and peace is the only thing of importance that is communicated. It is this attitude of the heart and not what is said between two people that does healing work in both directions. One party's accumulation of verbal knowledge is of little use to deep inner healing....

Love Is Our Essence.... The love in us can unite with the love in others, but two bodies cannot become one....

It is what we do with our hearts that affects others most deeply. It is not the movements of our body or the words within our mind that transmit love. We love from heart to heart....

A good rule for mental conduct is: think whatever makes you truly happy to think....

The mind can always be put to love rather than to one more review of what is already finished. Let bygones be bygones: let love be now....

[T]here is nothing in the material world as important as the love of God in our hearts. To allow a gradual and ever increasing release of that love is our only function.
—Gerald G. Jampolsky, M.D., *Teach Only Love*

"What is REAL?" asked the Rabbit one day, when they were lying side by side near the nursery fender, before Nana came to tidy the room. "Does it mean having things that buzz inside you and a stick-out handle?"

"Real isn't how you're made," said the Skin Horse. "It's a thing that happens to you. When a child loves you for a long, long time, not just to play with, but REALLY loves you, then you become real."

"Does it hurt?" asked the Rabbit.

"Sometimes," said the Skin Horse, for he was always truthful. "When you are Real you don't mind being hurt."

"Does it happen all at once, like being wound up," he asked, "or bit by bit?"

"It doesn't happen all at once," said the Skin Horse. "You become. It takes a long time. That's why it doesn't often happen to people who break easily, or have sharp edges, or have to be carefully kept. Generally, by the time you are Real, most of your hair has been loved off, and your eyes drop out and you get loose in the joints and very shabby. But these things don't matter at all, because once you are Real you can't be ugly, except to people who don't understand."
—Margery Williams, *The Velveteen Rabbit*

Chapter 11

Managing Stress

Just as water clarifies when you allow it to settle, the same is true with the mind.

—Lama Sogyal Rinpoche

TAKING CARE OF THE CAREGIVER

If you don't take care of yourself, then it is difficult to take care of others. If you are tired, cranky, or not feeling well emotionally or physically, you have nothing to give. You will feel drained and burnt out by continuing to give without replenishing your "self."

Whenever I tell someone I teach stress management, invariably the response is, "Boy, could I use that!" There are few of us who don't need it. By teaching I am also able to continually reinforce the techniques to better manage my own stress. Older people and people who care for older people are not exempt from life's stresses and may be in particular need of effective strategies for dealing with stress.

Stress comes from three basic sources: your environment, your body, and your thoughts. Environmental, emotional, and physical demands can cause your body to react to protect itself, and the nervous system reacts to protect you by creating what is called a "flight or fight" response. This is a primitive, inherited response that prepares us to fight or flee when we feel threatened. Stress as a mental process reveals itself in the body as muscle tension, backaches, anxiety, and fatigue. It reduces one's ability to concentrate, affecting the ability to think, work, learn, and relax. If you are continually stressed and the body is not given relief from these changes, chronic stress may result.

Chronic stress has been found to be related to a variety of ill-nesses, including high blood pressure, headaches, ulcers, coli-tis, arthritis, diarrhea, asthma, cardiac arrhythmias, sexual problems, circulatory problems, and muscle tension. By wear-ing you down, it can deteriorate you physically and emotional-ly as well as spiritualy.

There are innumerable classes and seminars in stress re-duction, and most people who participate get something out of them for the moment, and maybe for a short time after. How-ever, just as physical exercises that are done only once a month will not help your body feel in shape, stress management tech-niques done only occasionally will not benefit you. Stress is part of life, and each of us needs to take responsibility for our own responses to our stress. If you practice and integrate a few of these techniques into your everyday life, when a stressful situation arises it will be easier to deal with. Regular physical practices give the body strength, flexibility, and balance; regu-lar stress management practices can do the same for your emo-tional strength, flexibility, and balance.

This chapter is about how to use deep breathing as a relax-ation response and creative, fun body movement techniques to release stress; how to observe and refocus thought patterns; and how to utilize tools for self-expression, invoke humor, and tap into the strength of your inner self. Because each of us is different, I offer a variety of methods. Some are uniquely my invention and others are variations of more traditional tech-niques. Choose those that feel good, that you can commit to, and then integrate them into your life on a regular basis. My methods are practical, creative, and fun, and include a varied and eclectic approach. The experiential activities in this chap-ter are tools for living your joy, alleviating stress, and giving yourself permission to love yourself and therefore others.

Some years ago the *Washington Post* did an article about research that was done with people who lived past 100 years. It was thought that there would be a correlation to their life styles, such as eating and sleeping habits. What the researchers found instead was that these people had no such common fac-tors, but that there were six things they all did have in com-mon: *activity* (of some sort), *discipline* (for one man, it was nothing more than getting out of his pajamas and dressed every morning), *altruism* (helping one or more people), *optimism* (positive thinking), *spiritual faith* (of some kind), and *love of life.*

My belief is that the three major approaches to managing stress are: 1) quieting the mind and focusing with a relaxation technique, 2) some kind of physical activity—(my approach involves self-motivated, fun body movement and body awareness), and 3) being aware of and directing your own thoughts.

My prescription for managing stress is a balance of work, rest, exercise, play, good nutrition, sleep, friends who don't drain you, communication skills, creative outlets for self-expression, touch (hugs and massage), self-esteem, laughter, love, and a belief in a power higher than yourself (i.e., God, love, nature).

Only you can reduce your stress. What I share with you are the tools for managing stress. You make the choice of either using the tools or putting them away in a tool box, where they will do you no good. Find the tools in this chapter that you can commit to using regularly, that feel right for you. Some of these will only be appropriate for you as an individual and some may be appropriate for working with groups.

In order to start changing to a less stressful lifestyle, commit yourself to just one or two techniques. Don't delay. Care enough about yourself. You deserve it. Love yourself enough to give this to yourself. If you feel good about yourself, you will feel better about those you love and they will appreciate you even more. Remember to approach change with as much lightness and fun as you can, because life is too important to take too seriously.

QUIETING THE MIND: BREATHING AND FOCUSING

Breathing exercises can be done from 5 to 20 minutes at a time, one to three specific times a day, or at any time when you feel stressed or overwhelmed. When you are feeling overwhelmed or feeling a need for a break, it is important for you to give yourself permission to stop whatever it is you are doing and take a relaxation breathing break. Caregivers are often so busy taking care of everyone else that they forget to take care of themselves. Love yourself enough to care, to know you are worth it. Even if you have to lock yourself in a bathroom for a few minutes—*take the time.*

Smiling Inwardly

Sit down, uncross arms and legs, and relax. Take a very deep breath through your nose, filling your body with as much air as you can. When you exhale, empty out as much breath as you can. Inhale deeply again and, as you exhale, feel the breath wash through your body from your head all the way down and out your feet. Repeat and feel all the tension loosen, relax, melt away, and leave your body. Once more, as you breathe in, smile inwardly, feeling a very relaxed quality washing over you.

If you would like to, and can, repeat the process for a longer period of time, continuing to follow your breath from body part to body part down your body. If thoughts enter your mind, take note and let them wash away with the next breath. *Do not get attached to your thoughts.* Bring your attention back to your breathing—in and out, in and out. When you are ready, focus your attention on how your body is making contact with the chair (or floor if you are lying down). Then open your eyes, feeling refreshed and relaxed.

Sets of Five

This breathing exercise is described in detail in Chapter 8. Remember that breath is the bridge to life—breathe deeply and fully as you do this exercise. Concentrate on your breath and, if you become aware of any thoughts entering your mind, gently let go by bringing your attention back to your breath.

I Am Relaxed

A mantra is nothing more than the silent repetition of a word or a sentence that becomes your focus. The repetition helps to block out other thoughts that might occupy your mind and prevent you from relaxing mentally; it provides a brief "vacation" from stressful thinking and a specific point of concentration. A mantra does not have to be esoteric or from a language that is foreign to you. However, for some people, a foreign word may feel more romantic. Your particular mantra can be anything you choose, in any language, from a poem, a religious book, or any other source. It can be a short favorite saying; it can be something from your own religious background, such as a rosary or other prayer. It can be in any language you speak, perhaps one you grew up with if your parents or grandparents were from another country.

The following is a simple technique using the words "I am relaxed" as your mantra. Inhale as slowly and as deeply as you can and silently say to yourself, "I am." Then exhale just as deeply and fully, saying to yourself, "relaxed." You can repeat this process at least five times, or for as long as you would like to for up to 20 minutes.

SELF-MOTIVATED BODY MOVEMENT AND AWARENESS

Research shows that regular exercise helps alleviate tension and stress. Your body must be free before your mind can function to its fullest extent. The following activities are easy to do and take little time.

Circle, Stretch, and Shake

Using three words—*circle, stretch,* and *shake*—you can loosen and flex your joints and whole body and feel more awake and alive. You can do this exercise with or without music, inside or outside, sitting during parts of it, or standing and moving around. If you use music, choose music that motivates you and that you enjoy moving to. You may want to use different music for each of the movements.

Starting with your head, circle slowly a few times in each direction. After a few circles in each direction, you may quicken the pace if you'd like. Remember that for some people complete circles may be dangerous. Continue the process of circling each possible part of your body, moving down the body part by part—shoulders, arms, wrists, rib cage (if you can), torso, hips, legs, and ankles.

When you have completed circling, begin again at the top of your body and, moving down, stretch each body part in all directions. Be creative. Think of your body as a twist-tie or a pipe cleaner, making unusual shapes. Feel like a cat, tuning in to your body where it needs to, wants to, and feels good to stretch.

When you have completed stretching, shake out each and every part of your body, concluding with a whole body "shake." Now you will feel completely invigorated.

Body Part Dancing

Another fun body part warm-up and loosening activity is to do an improvisational dance with each part of your body. This is similar to the body part warm-up described in Chapter 4. Find music that appeals to you at the moment. Beginning at the top of your body, do a dance with your head, moving it in time with the music or with your own rhythm. Enjoy investigating the many different ways you can move your head as well as exploring the many ways it can move through space (up, down, back, under, etc.). When you feel finished with the "head dance," move down to another body part and do a dance with each until you feel that you have "greased" all your joints. You will feel warmer and looser; you have brought more oxygen into your lungs and circulated more of the blood in your body.

Kick the Can

An unusual yet fun way to increase energy and at the same time release anger and frustration is to kick the bottom part of a cookie can. This can be done holding the can in your hand from a sitting position, from a standing position while holding onto the back of a chair for support, or while walking across a room, stepping and kicking with one foot at a time. This activity is described more fully in Chapter 7.

Other Activities

You can choose any of the movement activities in this book that appeal to you to serve as self-motivated movement. If you enjoy any other physical activity, such as biking, tennis, running, dancing, or going to a gym, so much the better. Often I will spontaneously break into dance. This is not only a joy, but also a release of tension, a break from a serious, focused moment. My body is so accustomed to some form of physical activity that, if I don't do something physically active over a period of days, I feel awful. Sometimes, when I am travelling and am in a hotel, I use the steps as often as I can; this serves as a form of exercise that requires no special equipment or clothes to do.

DIRECTING YOUR THOUGHTS

Feeling/Thinking Check

Stressed people see everything as an immediate emergency. There is a saying about two men who looked through prison bars: One saw mud and the other saw stars. Where you choose to focus is your decision. Research has shown that people who are *"stress hardy"* have three "Cs" in their lives: Control (of self), Commitment, and Challenge. Another "C" that is undeniably important for all of us is Caring, which has to start with yourself. It has also been noted that those persons who survive change and loss the best are those who face these situations as a challenge.

Your perceptions, your focus, and your thoughts affect your feelings just as your feelings affect your thoughts. Some of us are aware that we are always talking to ourselves, and we never shut up—there is a constant dialogue going on that author Joseph Chilton Pearce called "roof brain chatter." What we are telling ourselves influences our experience of reality, our feelings and perceptions about what is going on. You are responsible for your thoughts. You can choose your attitude and your responses.

Begin to take note of your thoughts; become more aware. If you start to feel your mood change—an emotional state emerging—trace your thoughts for the last few minutes to see how your thinking may have exasperated the effects of a situation. It may take some effort for this to become habit, but the rewards will be worth it when you realize that you can, and do, have control over your thoughts.

Choosing Your Thoughts

Cognitive therapists Albert Ellis and David Burns have made a list of what they call irrational thoughts, or cognitive distortions, that dampen our feelings. Some of the distorted patterns of thought that can create stress and depression, according to Dr. Burns, are listed in Table 1.

A simple technique for stopping stressful thoughts is "reframing." One method of reframing is to put a rubber band on your wrist and, each time you become aware of obsessive, worrisome, or negative thoughts, gently snap the rubber band. Eventually, you won't need the rubber band, but will be able to

Table 1.   Definitions of cognitive distortions

1. ALL-OR-NOTHING THINKING: You see things in black-and-white categories. If your performance falls short of perfect, you see yourself as a total failure.

2. OVERGENERALIZATION: You see a single negative event as a never-ending pattern of defeat.

3. MENTAL FILTER: You pick out a single negative detail and dwell on it exclusively so that your vision of all reality becomes darkened, like the drop of ink that discolors the entire beaker of water.

4. DISQUALIFYING THE POSITIVE: You reject positive experiences by insisting they "don't count" for some reason or other. In this way you can maintain a negative belief that is contradicted by your everyday experiences.

5. JUMPING TO CONCLUSIONS: You make a negative interpretation even though there are no definite facts that convincingly support your conclusion.

   a. *Mind reading.* You arbitrarily conclude that someone is reacting negatively to you, and you don't bother to check this out.

   b. *The Fortune Teller Error.* You anticipate that things will turn out badly, and you feel convinced that your prediction is an already-established fact.

6. MAGNIFICATION (CATASTROPHIZING) OR MINIMIZATION: You exaggerate the importance of things (such as your goof-up or someone else's achievement), or you inappropriately shrink things until they appear tiny (your own desirable qualities or the other fellow's imperfections). This is also called the "binocular trick."

7. EMOTIONAL REASONING: You assume that your negative emotions necessarily reflect the way things really are: "I feel it, therefore it must be true."

8. SHOULD STATEMENTS: You try to motivate yourself with shoulds and shouldn'ts, as if you had to be whipped and punished before you could be expected to do anything. "Musts" and "oughts" are also offenders. The emotional consequence is guilt. When you direct should statements toward others, you feel anger, frustration, and resentment.

9. LABELING AND MISLABELING: This is an extreme form of overgeneralization. Instead of describing your error, you attach a negative label to yourself: "I'm a *loser.*" When someone else's behavior rubs you the wrong way, you attach a negative label to him: "He's a goddam louse." Mislabeling involves describing an event with language that is highly colored and emotionally loaded.

10. PERSONALIZATION: You see yourself as the cause of some negative external event which in fact you were not primarily responsible for.

From Burns, D.D. (1980). *Feeling good: The new mood therapy* (pp. 40–41). New York: William Morrow & Co.; reprinted by permission.

stop by just saying the word "stop," or by simply replacing the thought with another thought, poem, prayer, uplifting quote, or a positive mental image, such as a wonderful memory. You may want to choose one of the quotes provided here to use as your replacement thought of the week. You can pick another each week, or keep the same one until it no longer works for you.

The following quotations, uplifting thoughts, and reminders can be posted around your home and office. You can refer to them when you are feeling low, or obsessing with worrisome thoughts, or just need a nudge.

You gotta be a little crazy to keep from going insane.

—Unknown

Let yourself go loose occasionally and let yourself be silly.

A little craziness now and then could save you from permanent brain damage.

—Unknown

We either make ourselves miserable or make ourselves strong. The amount of work is the same.

—Carlos Castenada

Oh the comfort, the inexpressible comfort of being safe with a person, of having neither to weigh thoughts nor measure words. But pouring them all out chaff and grain together. Knowing that a faithful hand will receive them. Will keep what is worth keeping and with a breath of kindness blow the rest away!

—Shoshone Indian saying

Your interpretation of what you see and hear, is just that, your interpretation.

—Dr. Robert Anthony, *Think*

- *Whatever you assume to be true will become real for you.*
- *Life is what's coming, not what was.*
- *When it becomes more difficult to suffer than change…you will change.*
- *You will never "have it all together." That's like trying to eat once and for all!*

—Dr. Robert Anthony, *Think Again*

- *Wherever the mind goes, the energy flows.*
- *Your past is always going to be the way it was. Stop trying to change it.*

- *Argue long enough for your limitations, and they're yours.*
- *The road to success is always under construction.*
  —Dr. Robert Anthony, *Think On*

Life Lessons

1. *You will receive a body. You may like it or hate it, but it will be yours for the entire period this time around.*
2. *You will learn lessons. You are enrolled in a full-time informal school called life. Each day in this school you will have the opportunity to learn lessons. You may like the lessons or think them irrelevant and stupid.*
3. *There are no mistakes, only lessons. Growth is a process of trial and error: experimentation. The "failed" experiments are as much a part of the process as the experiment that ultimately "works."*
4. *A lesson is repeated until learned. A lesson will be presented to you in various forms until you have learned it. When you have learned it, you can then go on to the next lesson.*
5. *Learning lessons does not end. There is no part of life that does not contain its lessons. If you are alive, there are lessons to be learned.*
6. *"There" is no better than "here." When your "there" has become a "here" you will simply obtain another "there" that will, again, look better than "here."*
7. *Others are merely mirrors of you. You cannot love or hate something about another person unless it reflects to you something you love or hate about yourself.*
8. *What you make of your life is up to you. You have all the tools and resources you need, what you do with them is up to you. The choice is yours.*
9. *Your answers lie inside you. The answers to life's questions lie inside you. All you need to do is look, listen and trust.*
10. *You will forget all this.*

—Phoenix Services, Troy, Michigan

Finally, in a course I took with Christina Baldwin, author of *Life's Companion: Journal Writings as a Spiritual Quest* (1991), she suggested keeping a "Blessings Journal." At the end of each day, choose one blessing that occurred for you that day. A blessing can be something as simple as seeing the sunset, a call from a friend, or a meal you enjoyed. Whenever you are feeling low, look through your Blessings Journal and it will give you a lift.

Defining Directions in Your Life

As we grow older, whatever age we are, we often discover that, although our lives are full, our days seem to rush by with no opportunity to do many of the things we say we want to do "someday." Our lives seem out of focus and out of control, as though other people and events are moving us in directions we do not remember choosing. We realize our lives are being spent for us by others. Although it is important to be spontaneous and to let life flow, it is also important to have plans and goals, even in old age.

A great reminder and metaphor for focusing on what I *do* want, and where I *do* want to go, instead of what I don't, occurs for me when I bike along the pebbled towpath beside the old C&O canal. There are often large pebbles that I do not want to bike over, and I notice that, whenever I focus on one of those pebbles, I invariably go over it instead of avoiding it by focusing on where I *do* want to go.

The following techniques can be used to help give you focus and direction in your life, with a renewed sense of control and purpose.

Focusing on the Positive

From the book, *Living with Joy,* by Sanaya Roman (1986, pp. 109–110) come the following questions, which you can give yourself as an assignment:

1. What do you appreciate having in your life right now?
2. Whom do you appreciate having, or whom have you had in your life?
3. What things about yourself—body, mind, etc.—do you appreciate?
4. Call or write someone you like that you have not been in touch with for at least a year.

Setting Priorities

Time management is one of the *big* stressors. Make a list of *your* priorities and then keep a journal of how you spend each minute of your day. You can then see what you can eliminate, or at least limit, such as telephone time and television time (unless, of course, these are on your list of stress reducers!). But here again, it is your responsibility to choose and number your priorities, making sure you balance work and play in your choices.

First read the following poem.

Before I Go

Before I go, I'd like to have high cheekbones.
I'd like to talk less like New Jersey, and more like
   Claire Bloom
And whenever I enter a room, I'd like an orchestra
   to burst into my theme song.
I'd like to have a theme song before I go.

Before I go, I'd like to learn to tap dance.
I'd like to play seven-card stud like a pro, not
   a dunce.
And I'd like Robert Redford, just once, to slide his
   fingers down my back from my neck to my waistline.
I'd like to have a waistline before I go.

Before I go, I'd like to win the door prize.
I'd like to be thought of as valiant and brilliant and thin.
And I'd like, when offered a choice between duty and sin,
   to not immediately choose duty.
I'd like a couple of offers before I go.

Before I go, I'd like to make things better.
I'd like to be told I've been more of a joy than a pain.
And I'd like those I love to know that they are the ones,
   if I could do it again, I'd do it with.
I'd like to do it again before I go.

                                        —Judith Voirst, *Forever 50*

   After reading this poem (with humor), write the words "Before I go," and make your own serious list of what you want to do and have before you go. Writing is more powerful than just doing it in your head. The process of writing will help you become more aware of your desired directions.

Choosing to Laugh

Do not feel totally, personally, irrevocably, responsible for everything. That is my job. Love, God

                                        —Unknown

Life is too important to take so seriously. Humor is a great releaser of stress. Joel Goodman, director of the Humor Project in Saratoga Springs, New York, states that, "Research shows that laughing inhibits stress hormones, and studies have shown that people with a good sense of humor are more successful without being more stressed."

A fun way to alleviate a stressful situation is to blow it out of proportion. Allen Elkin, Ph.D., program director of Stresscare Systems, Inc., calls this the "blow-up method."

> It's a tension diffuser that involves blowing up a situation to the point of ludicrousness. It can make you laugh and diffuse a volatile situation. Here's how it works. Let's say you're in a traffic jam. Bumper-to-bumper. Instead of fuming in silence, talk out the most horrible scenario you can imagine. I'll be stuck here for hours. These cars will *never* move. They'll have to close the freeway and airlift us out of here. Of course, they'll probably have one helicopter to airlift thousands of cars. By the time they get to me, my children will have grown up, married and had children of their own. No one will even remember who I am. (1989, p. 42)

By imagining the worst-case scenario, "to the point of absurdity, you begin to smile to yourself" and let go of catastrophizing (Elkins, 1989, p. 42).

Norman Cousins, in his book, *Anatomy of an Illness as Perceived by the Patient* (1979), tells how he used regular sessions of laughter as part of his healing from a serious illness. Before his death, he taught a course about positive emotions in healing to medical students. In an essay he wrote for *The Age-less Spirit*, he stated, "I've always regarded laughter as a metaphor for the full range of the positive emotions, of which I would certainly include hope and faith and love and will to live, determination, purpose, and creativity" (1992, p. 45). How many times a day do you have a good belly laugh? Find ways to laugh, and people with whom you can do this often.

PART III

SELF-EXPRESSION
THROUGH THE ARTS

Chapter 12

Ideas for Creating Poetry and Recording Oral History

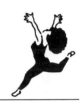

If I had my life to live over again, I would make it a rule to read some poetry and listen to some music at least once every week. The loss of these tastes is a loss of happiness.

—Charles Darwin

Because my background and training are in dance, and my focus starts with the body, when I do an activity that involves other forms I usually start with movement. There are other times, however, when I might begin with music, art, or poetry. Older adults enjoy the creative processes. Many have never had the opportunity to explore their creativity in the arts. A few may feel silly or intimidated at times, but, most often, once they start, they do get involved. One study of a group of 70-year-olds at the University of California showed that, as the subjects grew older, they demonstrated increasing diversity and uniqueness (Maas & Kuypers, 1974).

Being creative taps into some of the childlike qualities and our ability to let go and play. Staying in touch with the child within us is important throughout life. Mencius, who lived in China in the fourth century B.C., said: "A great person is one who never loses the heart of a child." And Jesus said, "Only children can enter the Kingdom of Heaven."

Ronald Manheimer, Director of the National Council on Aging's Humanities Program, writes,

> There is a magical, sometimes fearful, sensation to creativity because one is, in a sense, reinventing the world. While there is a strong element of play, it is play accompanied by a deep serious-ness and sense of risk. Creative experiences expand the person's perceptions.... Creativity...can empower a person to take greater initiative in all areas of life and to find bonds of solidarity with peers. (1986)

PERSPECTIVES AND COMMUNICATION

Before I start a creative process, I sometimes talk about how we see things, our varied perspectives, how difficult communica-tion can be, how we interpret what we hear and what we see, and how the arts can be a means for communication. I begin with a story about communication and expectation:

> A man receives a letter saying he will receive a gift of a chair in the mail. In his mind, he envisions a carved wood, tufted velvet, thronelike chair and gets very excited. He can hardly wait for the chair to arrive and, when it finally does, he finds it is a folding metal chair.

Given that we all speak the same language, we assume that a simple, everyday word like "chair" can easily be under-stood. I ask the group to close their eyes and visualize the first chair that comes to their mind. I then ask each to describe his or her chair and maybe share a story about the chair, if it was one that had personal meaning to them. Some just describe a chair like: "a beach chair," "a bench," "an ice cream parlor chair," and so on. I ask each to describe the chair in detail (i.e., what kind of wood, metal, fabric, color, or other material). I ask them to be as specific as they can. Often, there are only two chairs that are alike or similar in a group of 30 or more people. Others provide stories about chairs that were "the one that was in my home as I grew up," "the one my dad always sat in," and "the one I fed (or nursed) my children in." These kinds of de-scriptions let the group learn a more personal piece of informa-tion about this person's life.

A discussion follows about our different perceptions based on our diverse backgrounds, and how communication is not easy—how misunderstanding or misinterpretation can evolve. I then read a few haikus (short poems of Japanese origin) one at a time, and ask the group to close their eyes, listen, and allow their minds to picture images. Then I ask them to share their images for each poem. Realization of our different perceptions is discussed, reminding us that *all* are correct; there are no "wrong" answers. What we perceive is our reality.

WRITING HAIKU

When I work with mentally alert older adults who might like to be mentally challenged, like the groups at Elderhostel, I often use the Japanese poetry style called haiku. Depending on the ability of the group, I may read the rules of writing a haiku. The poem consists of three lines: The first line contains five syllables; the second line, seven syllables; and the third line, five syllables. In a haiku, there is usually a name of a season or a key word to imply it, a reference to nature, and a feeling. There is implied identity between two different things. I tell the group that this is just the jumping-off point and that the rules *do not* have to be adhered to, that there are no grades and whatever they write will be acceptable.

I am continually excited by the creativity that comes out in *every* group. The following are a few samples from a group at Elderhostel at Columbia Union College, October 1987:

Dark and stormy clouds
Wind and rain race overhead
Come see the rainbow
   —Peggy Askoff

Blue skies, autumn flowers blooming
Sunshine casting shadows
 in lacy patterns
Soft, cool breezes, blowing gently.
     —Ruta

Time Is Now
Enjoy Enjoy
Enjoy Enjoy
Enjoy
Life is short.
—Pearl Lanotzl

Elderhostel

No, not so elder
And certainly not hostel
Help, please call Boston.
                —Evelyn Griffith

I usually tell the group that the point is to express themselves. I am not concerned if the haiku rules are broken.

Some participants are inspired to explore other types of poetry. The following poem was influenced by our haiku session at Elderhostel at Columbia Union College (C.U.C.):

Our Week at C.U.C.

Listen my children and you shall hear,
What we did at Elderhostel this year.
From Columbia Union in Takoma Park
We bused to the capital like beasts in the ark.

We came to Washington, D.C.
Its many monuments to see.
Washington, Lincoln and Jefferson too,
The Marian Shrine at Catholic U.
The National Cathedral in Gothic design,
Of course, the Capitol with dome so fine.

I traced the name of my stepson tall,
Engraved upon the Vietnam wall.
In the Space Museum and African Hall,
I learned a lot and had a ball.

We observed computers of many brands,
At simple programming we tried our hands.
We exercised and wrote haiku,
All our tensions to undo.

This was in the seat of the nation,
It has been a capital vacation!
                —Barbara Hussey Riggins

A Multi-arts Process

I use haiku as a foundation for an integrated arts process, focusing on communication and interpretation. First I ask the class to write individual haikus. When they have completed the writing of their poems, I ask everyone to do a drawing—realistic or abstract—that depicts the poem. When each person has done his or her own poem, has read it to the group, and has shared his or her drawing, I ask small groups of three to six people whose poems' subject matter is similar to come together to create one poem. I tell them that they have creative license and can put their poems together in any way they like, including putting them all together, stanza by stanza, to make one poem, or they can take one line from each poem to make one poem, or any other way they can come up with. The next part of this process is to add sound effects and music. The sound effects can be a hissing sound done by the whole group to represent the wind, rattling paper to sound like leaves, bells to represent birds, or a rhythmic clapping of hands as a background. Music can be made using musical instruments or a tape of one or more pieces of music. I tell the group they can use any of the musical instruments or tapes that I have with me.

Each group can then create their own dance or movement, and put the whole thing together using their drawings and musical accompaniment. If one person does not wish to dance, he or she can do the reading or play the instruments. The performing group can even ask the rest of the group to do the reading or the music. If a group is stuck, I offer my help or input, but this is seldom needed.

When the process is complete, or after a given amount of limited time, each group presents theirs to the rest of the groups. I tell them this is not an artistic venture, but just a quick and fun way of practicing creativity. I have always had every group come up with something, and usually they are funny, creative, and sometimes quite beautiful.

Haiku and Other Poetry for Facilitators

I include poetry in my teacher training, staff development, and stress management courses and workshops as well. Not only is this a creative means of self-expression, but it acts as an initiator for sharing and social interactions and stretches the participants to use their minds in ways they usually don't. It also gives them the chance to speak or perform before a group. For some this is fun and for some it is scary. All learn that they can do it.

In a course I teach at the University of Maryland, five students put their haikus together as follows:

The dawn of the early morning
brings the sunlight to the world
and the love of a young child's touch.

The sun shines, brightly
Warmth, splendor, light giving life
how fortunate—us.

The wilderness is sought
to enjoy the peaceful and calm
and reflect on life.

As quiet snow falls
on the earth sleeping below
the world is at peace.

The moon, the stars are
soothing, peaceful, and calming.
I am refreshed.
—Theresa, Gary, Eileen, Ron, and Jim

In this same class I asked the group to call out their thoughts and perceptions of rain while I wrote them down:

Rain

Leaky basements
   cold
Refreshing
   Spring
Noisy pitter patter
Washes away the dirt
Torrential downpour
   and the smell before the rain

Pink umbrella, red galoshes
Blue raincoat
and rainbows.

At a recent therapy conference in Milwaukee, where I presented a workshop, one of the participants wrote the following haiku:

The lake is grayness
Big as an ocean blue
Yet its own child as well.
             —Maynard

No matter what kind of group I work with or what my approach is with each, I believe in the combined approach of body, mind, and spirit. Although I am not a trained teacher of English or poetry, I am a trained movement educator who has a feel for sound, rhythm, and creative self-expression. All things dance for me—the movements of nature, objects, music, and words.

WRITING GROUP POETRY AND ORAL HISTORY

Group Poetry

In many cases, it is easier to ask the group to create poetry *as a group*, with each person contributing some words or a line that I write. This method of creating poetry is more appropriate for those who cannot write or spell, or for frail or confused older people, and can be fun for any group. I write the words and sentences down as they are spoken. By taking dictation, there is less intimidation because of handwriting or spelling. Also, for those who have poor eyesight or shaky hands, or are otherwise physically unable to write, there is no separation of the group into the "can"s and "cannot"s. I do not change the words or the order in which they are dictated to me. Occasionally, I reorganize some of the lines so that there is an order or progression of ideas and thoughts. Occasionally, I repeat one word or one sentence for rhythm or dramatic effect, but for the most part I do not tamper with any part of what and how the words are expressed.

During group poetry writing, experiences are shared and there is more social interaction. What each person says, and how it is said, is valued and considered important. One contribution precipitates another, just like a brainstorming session. At the completion of each poem, both the group and each individual feel a pride of accomplishment.

When I lead classes in the creation of group poetry, most often I choose a subject, such as a rainy day, chairs, a full moon, favorite colors, or summertime, and ask for words and sentences expressing ideas, feelings, and memories about this chosen subject. I say, "Tell me what comes to your mind when you think of summertime." Other ideas for stimulating poetry or verbal sharing are:

- Halloween
- Thanksgiving
- Christmas
- Birthdays
- Things I wish I'd done
- Vacations I have taken
- Places I've been
- Smells, sights, sounds, and tastes of summer, winter, spring, or fall
- First day of school

With frail or confused persons, more prodding and specific direction often is needed. I am able to get a response from even very frail and confused participants or those who rarely respond. One of the subjects I like to use in these groups is "Favorite Colors." I just go to each person and ask, "What is your favorite color?" and then I ask, "Why?" I follow up this question with, "What things are this color?"

The following is an excerpt from such a poem that was created by a group of very frail and confused older adults at Hillhaven Nursing Center:

My Favorite Color Is:

Yellow, because daisies and sunshine are yellow.
Red; I like it because it bleached your hair.
  Apples, some pears and cherries are red.
Green; I don't know why,
  I just think it's good!
Pale blue, because I have blue eyes.
  Part of my skirt is blue.
Purple, because some kinds of grapes are purple.
  Pansies are purple and it's royal.
Rose, because my name is Rosalie.
  A dress I have and some flowers are rose.
Green, because so many different shades
  of nature are green,
  like leaves of trees, flowers and the grass.

Writing this poem initiated a response, a presence, a process of thinking and communicating these thoughts, as well as putting the participants in touch with awareness, feelings, and some memories. This is helpful because these frail and confused older adults are usually very inward, and sometimes irritable, and often resist response to activities.

This same group wrote a poem on another subject I suggested, summertime:

Summertime

It's hot as hell!
Swimming
   and cleaning up and
   cut the grass.
It's HOT!
It breezes.
Warm weather and ice cream and picnics.
Go out in the country and enjoy it.
When you get old
   all the things in your mind go away.
      And now time is in my mind.

I think the last three lines of this poem are particularly expressive.

Something as simple as the moon was the subject for this poem, written by a group at the Evelyn I. Cole Multipurpose Senior Center:

The Moon

The sky
I think of light
I wonder if it's a blue moon or an orange moon?
Is it true that there's a man in the moon?
Or does it just appear to be?
Full Moon, Silver Moon, Harvest Moon, Hot Moon
The population increases on the full moon
Bride soon, Honeymoon too
Half Moon, Quarter Moon and Crescent Moon too.

The following poem was written by participants at the Greater Southeast Community Center for the Aging Saturday Program for deinstitutionalized clients with mental illness from St. Elizabeth's Hospital:

My Favorite Things

Playing records to my poetry
Buying clothes, buying clothes

Cooking
Watching TV
Shopping for holly at the five and ten cent store
Shopping for skirts at Marianne
Eating ice cream
Listen to the FM station all day
Shopping for groceries, especially fruit at the
    Safeway or Giant.

At one adult day care center at the University Fellowship Club, in which the group featured a variety of mental and physical abilities, the members needed a lot of prodding. The following is an excerpt from one of their poems:

Halloween

I think you got to be careful
    who comes to your door
Witches, skeletons, cats, goblins
    and pumpkin pies.

I often use a holiday or a season as the subject of the poem, such as Thanksgiving, Christmas, Martin Luther King Day, or spring or fall. When I use a holiday or season as the subject, I ask for any memories, thoughts, ideas, or feelings about the particular holiday or season. If there is no response, I will start by telling one of my thoughts. Or I ask a specific question, like, "Do you remember any specific Thanksgiving?" "What do you do on Thanksgiving?" "What do you eat?" "What are you thankful for?" As soon as one person starts, others follow and thoughts and memories pour out. The following is an example of a poem written about Martin Luther King Day by a group at the Cole Senior Center:

Martin Luther King Remembered

Peace for all men.
Love for all mankind.
Nonviolence, courage, determination.
Religious dedication, gratitude.
He had a dream and he followed it.
He taught us all tolerance.
He was a Christian in the truest sense of the word.
He had conviction and passion for his beliefs.
His words to the world would be:
LOVE, PEACE, JUSTICE, BROTHERHOOD and UNITY.

My approach in working with groups is to focus on the positive—not to ignore the negative, but to look at the glass as half full rather than half empty. As in the poem "Ithaca," by C.P. Cavefy, when you "anchor at the isle when you are old, rich with all that you have gained on the way," my approach is to motivate the good memories along the way to the mythical Ithaca.

After a group has had the experience of writing a poem and has the feeling of success, I usually ask for more than just a memory or thought. In a poem about happiness, I asked a group at the Hillhaven Nursing Center to think about the sound, the feel, and the color of happiness. The following is an excerpt from one of these poems:

Happiness

Happiness is walking through the woods
   hearing the birds singing
   and the trees saying whoosh, whoosh, whoosh.
Happiness is snuggling down in bed
   just before you go to sleep.
Riding horseback through the woods;
   I could do that forever!
My first wagon and
   Flexible Flyer sled—
   Crunch, shhh, crunch, shhh
     Wheeeeeee.
The color of happiness is pink
   like pink clouds,
   because I always feel good when
   I look at pink.
   It's such a soft sweet color.
The color of happiness is blue
   because it's a soothing color
   and it's pretty like a sunset
   or a clear, blue sky.

When trying to extend the thought process beyond the literal, I might suggest analogies or metaphors. Here are some excerpts from "Emotions Are Like," by a group at the Hillhaven Nursing Center:

A soft white cloud
   is like a peaceful dream.
A frisky puppy is like
   a happy day.

Beautiful music
   is like flowing dance.
The soft strings of a violin
   are like love.
A thunderstorm
   is like war.
Lightning is like a beautifully lit
   Christmas tree.
Gently flowing small streams,
   in the woods
   are like tranquility
   and are comforting.
A racing horse trotting to the finish line
   is like a train going down the hill,
   is like looking into the future
   with excitement.
A soft baby kitten
   is like a train whistle in the night
   which is like lonesome feeling.
The shaking of the leaves on the trees
   is like Jell-O and is like
   being nervous and scared
The group from Hillhaven's Nursing Center outing to
   the restaurant for lunch reminded me of
   a family reunion which is
   joyous with talking and laughter.

Because a great part of my classes are focused on movement, I sometimes like to use subjects that motivate us to move, poems we can move with, such as, "Things That Go Round" and "Things That Move." These stretch the imagination as well as the body.

All movement begins with breath. I often bring in props that initiate different kinds of breathing, such as candles to blow out, pinwheels, and soap bubbles (see Chapter 1). After doing these activities, it is interesting to have the participants share memories of other things they have blown. Here are some from one such group:

Blowing

I remember blowing up a balloon for one of my young children and it broke. He ran around the room looking for it and crying, "Where did it go, where did it go?"

I blew out gas lights.

When I was little, I used to love to blow
on dandelion fluff, the seeds.
We called it the dandelion clock and after blowing
you count the seeds that are left
and that's what time it is.

I remember my uncle took me to an outdoor dance and
he brought me purple balloons that my mom blew up for
me when I got home, and the next day they had deflated.
I cried and cried until we went out and bought new ones.

I remember blowing out the coal oil lamps
before we went to bed.

I enjoy stimulating people with new experiences and
stretching their thoughts, which can then be put into a poem. I
often bring in ideas or objects that will influence these, such as
a multiprism lens. Because I usually dress in bright colors and
outrageous earrings, I often hear someone saying, "What is she
wearing today?" I have an enormous collection of very big,
very long, unusual clip-on earrings, and one day I brought them
all in. I had the residents of the nursing home choose the ones
they wanted to try on and then I walked around with some
hand mirrors so that they could see themselves. Photos were
taken as well. The following are excerpts from the poem that
came out of this experience:

Earrings

Feels like a party.
I feel like a different person, more daring.
I feel like I'm going out dancing.
I'm not used to them—to tell you the truth
   I don't know how I feel.
I feel like I'm all dressed up and
   ready to go among people,
   not ordinary people,
   but movie stars and celebrities.
I'm not ashamed to go among the best people.
All dressed up and no place to go.
I wear them all the time,
   but these are different—
   they're longer—nuttier!
I feel all dressed up.
I feel like a madam—
   Madam X—she was BAD.

Here are some excerpts from poems about my classes:

We laugh and have lots of fun
    and sometimes we groan too.
And sometimes she brings in:
    A happiness to my life.
    Talking teddy, drum bear,
    Skating bear, scarves, drums,
    Sticks and kick the cookie can.
We're on stage because people stop to look
    on their way by.
We swing and sway with Pauline.
We hug our knees and we wiggle everything in here.
We enjoy ourselves, we have fun.
This is the most fun we have.
We end all our classes with being silly and
    a happy hug and LOVE.
                    —Hillhaven Nursing Center

Class is invigorating, challenging and makes me feel good.
My body is tingling.
I love Pauline because she has extended my life.
Bending, stretching, jumping, running, walking
    Dancing, Dancing, Dancing.
We're stiff when we come in and we go out limber.
I love the way we end our classes,
    cooling down with hugs and love
    and our friendship circle.
Communicating through our silent prayers.
                    —Cole Senior Center

On one occasion, I arrived at the Cole Senior Center apologetic because I had forgotten to come and do a make-up class the day before, something I'd never done before. As it was, no one else remembered either. We decided to write the following poem:

Forgetting

Yesterday, I was supposed to go to the doctor at
    Two and I went at Ten.
I always forget where I park my car.
I came all the way home from work and realized that
    I had left my purse there.
Once I left my bag at the security check of an airport,
    but when I went back it was still there.

I was supposed to be at church at 11:30 to meet with
   a group that I had started and I got there at 12 instead.
I forgot to pay my AT&T bill in December.
I forgot my anniversary.
One day, I went out and forgot to close my front door;
   I left it wide open.
I went grocery shopping this morning, got to the checkout and
   realized I didn't have my courtesy card,
   but the manager had mercy on me and
   let me cash my check.
Last week, I did the same thing,
   I had forgotten my checkbook,
   but they let me pile it all up and held it for me.
I did the same thing, I had forgotten my Social Security card.
I took the wrong car to get seat belts put on
   and didn't realize it until I got there.
I wore my shirt inside out and didn't know it.
If I said all the things I forgot, it would make a whole book.

This turned out to be a healing process, cathartic for us all. Since that time, I have had groups express themselves and put into a poem our feelings, thoughts, and memories at the death of a group member, or a resignation of a staff member. We also make a poem card when a group member is sick or hospitalized.

Oral History

The importance of oral history is now being recognized. There is a natural inclination for reviewing one's life and for sharing it with others. This serves to acknowledge to the self and others, "I was here." Participating in group poetry gives everyone the opportunity to tell parts of his or her personal history. It also helps to stimulate memories of the past, and to relive events both old and recent. When the groups I visit on a regular basis have gone on an outing, I ask them to tell me about it so we can put the memories into a poem. This gives them a chance to share the experiences and relive them and gives me a chance to be a part of the group.

Subjects that I have used to initiate memories have been "Family Fun," "Favorite Foods," and "Sights and Smells and Tastes of Summer." For the first of these, I asked what kinds of things their families had done as a group to have fun. A group at the Hillhaven Nursing Center wrote the following poem:

My mother and father used to sit by the Latrobe*
   and tell us stories and my father would
   make them up as he went along. He'd also
   play the mandolin and make lots of
   mistakes and make a face.

My grandmother used to sit at her spinning wheel
   and we would listen to her stories about
   princes and princesses.

We used to crack walnuts.
We made fudge.
We pulled taffy—
   the more we pulled the lighter it got
   until it got hard.

[*A kind of pot belly stove]

Food is such an important part of each day for nursing
home residents, because it's one of the few main events of the
day. I thought talking about it would be enjoyable. What I got,
however, were memories from the past of food as it related to
home and warm feelings, and these led to thoughts and words
about more of the senses. Here are some excerpts from a poem
by a group at the Hillhaven Nursing Center:

Black raspberry pie that my mother made;
   we only had at raspberry time
   when I would go and pick the raspberries.
My own chicken dumplings;
   I probably forgot how to make them
   it's been so long.
My own fruit cake reminds me of Christmas.
   I used to make one for everybody in
   my family and started the day after
   Thanksgiving.
I liked everything Mom made
   and what comes to mind now is
   her citrus and other fruit marmalades
   that we used to put on toast or anything.
   It was gorgeous to look at and
   delicious to taste.
Mashed potatoes with gravy
   I always ate as a child.
   One time we were in Philadelphia at a hotel,
   when I was a child and I asked for

mashed potatoes and the waitress said,
"We don't have any." I said,
"Well go mash some!"
Apple pie without the cheese is like a kiss without
the squeeze.

The group at Hillhaven also wrote a poem on summer:

The Sights and Smells and Tastes of Summer

The slap of a fish as he jumps in and out of the water.

The candy shops down by the boardwalk—
salt water taffies and popcorn,
snow cones and Planter's peanuts,
cotton candy and ice cream cones.

The spray of the water as a boat passes.
The harsh sound of a fog horn.
The flight of the cranes.

Hosing off the front porch in your bathing suit.
The sweet smell of damson and grape jelly
boiling on the stove before canning
And blackberry wine anytime you want it.

Two of my favorite poem subjects have been "I Remember" and "Things We Used to Have That We Don't Have Now." Older adults have a wealth of memories, and focusing on these subjects is a wonderful way to bring those memories to the surface, to give them an opportunity for sharing and an outlet for creative expression. I believe the excerpts from the following poems speak for themselves.

I Remember

When things were very good.
I remember when my four-year-old daughter went into my closet
and tried to cut the roses out of my blue dress
I remember getting a pair of scissors
and cutting off my sister's curls
I'm not telling what I got afterwards.
I remember when my father took me to the circus
and gave me a peanut to give to the elephant,
but when the elephant reached
I got frightened and pulled the peanut back.
At this the elephant put his trunk
into the mud and let me have it!

As a youngster in Austria, the boys and girls
    walked to the meadows in the mountains
    and picked edelweiss from under the snow.
I remember Pearl Harbor.
I remember getting spanked and saying,
    "I'm gonna spit my gum out
    on your blue and white apron."
    And for that I got an extra spank.
I remember watching my brother and his friend play tennis
    I wanted to play,
    but they wouldn't let me,
    so I never learned.
I remember getting my teeth checked at school
    and the dentist pulled one of my teeth.
    I think he was practicing on me,
    learning how to pull teeth on a poor kid!
                            —Hillhaven Nursing Center

I remember my wedding day.
I remember the last 11 months and
    how bad I've been wanting to come to this center.
I remember the beautiful aromas
    that came from my mother's kitchen
    especially this time of the year
    when she was baking bread, pies and other goodies.
I remember when I was small and it snowed;
    during the second snow storm we would go out and get snow
    and make ice cream snow cream
    with sugar, cream, and vanilla flavoring.
I remember my mother's beautiful long black hair
    and how I would braid it when I was about 9.
    She died before I was 10.
    I missed her so much, and still do.
I remember my dear grandmother, Margerite,
    the love she had for me
    and the fun we had together.
    I went to her house every day
    and she gave me everything I wanted.
I remember one Sunday morning
    in the early spring when I was a child,
    I went out to pick violets and the sun was shining so bright.
    It was such a beautiful day and such a happy time in my life.
    I've never forgotten it.
I remember the bedtime stories my mother used to read to us
    by the lamplight and my father was as much a child
    and was just as interested as we were.
    She read from Grimm's Fairy Tales and

Uncle Remus and Cinderella and much more.
I remember when I was 15 and was baptized
    and such a spiritual feeling came over me and into my heart.
    I learned how to pray and I felt close to the Lord.

—Cole Senior Center

I remember when I cut my sister's curls off,
    they were down to her knees.
My sister took me into the back yard
    and cut each of my long curls one at a time.
    My father grabbed all her curls in one hand
    and was going to cut them off—
    but he changed his mind.
I remember when I dressed the dog up.
I remember when I was about 6
    I stole into my father's wine closet and drank some wine.
    I fell asleep behind the couch and they called the police
    because they couldn't find me,
    until someone moved the couch
    and I rolled from under.
      Then I came near getting a whipping,
But they were so happy to see me I didn't get one.
I remember my army serial number—RH22921045.
I remember when I was a very young child and I'm 90 now.
    My father raised little baby chicks and I loved them so
    I squeezed them to death—
    My father couldn't imagine why all those chicks were dying,
    until one day, when he caught me and scolded me so.
    So many things I could have remembered,
    especially at this age,
    but this seems to be the most outstanding memory.

—Manor Care Nursing Home

Things We Used to Have That We Don't Have Now

A Ferris waist gave you a nicer shape and held up your stockings.
    We started wearing them at about 13, when we started wearing
    bras, or when you had something to put in them (or hoped to).
    Later they were made more like corsets.
We used to have the side garters and then the roll-up kind.
    Now we have pantyhose and knee and thigh highs.
In the '20s we had dance marathons and now there's
    rock and roll dancing on TV.
We used to have the Depression and World War I.
    Veterans used to sell apples at a nickel apiece.
    Used to buy a little bunch of flowers for about 15 cents
    The veterans sold poppies and the money went for charity.
You don't see horses in the garage anymore.
    and don't have to clean up after them either.

I remember the rats we wore to wrap our hair around.
I remember when a penny could buy something.
I remember polio.
I remember the days of quarantine—
  with scarlet fever and diphtheria.
How about the old trolley cars?
    Put 50 cents away so you'd have carfare for a week.
    They had a motorman who drove
    and halfway down the car
    was a conductor who collected your fare.
I remember hobble skirts; they were real tight
    with a five-inch slit up the back so you could walk.
    "Hobble hobble little maid, wonder you're not afraid!"
A horse and buggy and baby buggies.
High-button shoes and the button hook.
Middie blouses and snuggies.
Washboards and washtubs.
Clothes pins and clothes lines.
There used to be swimming holes
    that the boys had and went naked,
    but we girls were not allowed.
I remember the lamplighter. He had a ladder
    and a long pole that he could reach up with.
Before electric and gas, we used coal and wood
    and so we needed chimney sweeps.
    They had black high hats, black suits like an evening coat
    and carried an assortment of brooms.
    Their faces were black from the soot.
    It frightened us children; we ran like 60!
Movies used to be a nickel and we stayed all afternoon.
    They had a piano player for the silent films.
And in the winter time when there was a rain puddle that froze,
    we used to go skating, but mostly on the seat of our pants.
                                    —Hillhaven Nursing Center

The memories evoked by these poems—not just for the things that are missed but for parts of the self that have been lost or never developed—are sad, funny, warm, and picturesque, and reveal bits of nostalgia, I learned about things I had never heard of before from the last poem, as well as expressions used years ago, such as "dainties" and "run like 60." I was interested to find that cutting off sister's curls came up so often.

When a comment is made in the group that I think will make a good trigger for a poem, I say, "That's a good title for our next poem." For example, when I brought photos from a recent vacation to show to the residents of a nursing home, one woman exclaimed, "Oh, I wish I had traveled more; I would have gone to Hawaii and danced the hula." I told her we would find a way that she could still dance the hula. Maybe we could all contribute to a poem about things we didn't do, but wished we had. We could follow this poem with one about things we did do and wished we hadn't. The following are poems written just as the group expressed themselves:

Things I Didn't Do That I Wish I Had Done

I wanted to go to Hawaii and I never got there.
    I would have put on a grass skirt and danced the hula.
I never roller skated.
I always wanted to go to the Netherlands,
    but had no way to get there—
        I couldn't swim.
I would have liked to get on a big hill on a sled
    to see how far I could go
        without falling off.
I wish I could have gone to a New York first-class restaurant.
I wish I could have gone on the stage—
    a real stage in New York—to act.
I wish I had done cartwheels.
Don't you wish you had visited every country in the world
    and put on their costumes?
I've never been in an airplane.
                        —Hillhaven Nursing Center

Things I Didn't Do That I Wish I Had

I regret that I didn't finish college and get at least two degrees.
I wish I had learned to swim.
I didn't continue my piano lessons and I wish I had.
I wish I had visited my mother more
    than I did while I still could.
I wish I had finished my driving lessons.
I wish I had finished school.
I wish I had entered high school, which I didn't.
I wish I hadn't gotten married so soon so I could
    have become a professional singer.
        Some wealthy people offered to back me
        to be a movie star and I didn't accept,
        I wish I had.
I wish I had entered a class to be a nurse's aide.
I wish I had been a president of the United States.
                        —Cole Senior Center

Things I Did and Wish I Hadn't

When I was real little I put my finger on the screen on what
 I thought was a fly, but it was a bee and it stung me.
I wish I hadn't married my first husband.
I wish I had never gotten sick.
I wish I hadn't stopped smoking; I still desire it.
I wish I hadn't given my car away.
When I was a little girl, I saw a little hole in the ground and
 I put my finger in it and felt a pinch—
 when I pulled it out, there was a mouse hanging on my finger.
I wish I hadn't gained so much weight as I have.
I wish I hadn't burned a hole in my skirt.
I wish I hadn't stopped practicing the piano,
 because now I can't play.

—Hillhaven Nursing Center

For those groups in the nursing home, this was a way of expressing and releasing, or at least sharing, some feelings. Some of the "Wish I hads" can be done in mime and made into a dance, such as dancing the hula, roller skating, and swimming. You could even talk about and then mime dining in a New York first-class restaurant, bringing in photos and menus. At a later time, I did bring in a hula skirt and hula music, so each could dance the hula. I was even able to wrap it around those persons using wheelchairs.

For those groups in recreation centers or similar facilities, these revelations help them see that, if they really wanted to do these things, they could still do them. The ones they couldn't do, they could at least let go of by expressing and sharing.

Chapter 13

Fun Activities
for Creating Art

*Intuition is your guide here. One level of you knows
everything there is to know. Find that level, ask for guidance,
and trust you'll be led wherever you most need to go. Try it.*
—Richard Bach, *One*

E xpressing one's self through abstract art or realistic
drawing is not only a means of communication, but
can be calming or even stimulating. Sometimes words do not
express our feelings, or even our meanings, satisfactorily, but
by drawing we can often express a deeper part of our psyche.
We don't have to understand what we have drawn to feel grati-
fied. The drawing may express what we felt symbolically or
metaphorically. Using colors and a variety of art supplies can
stimulate creativity and excite the mind, triggering new ideas.
Or, the colors and the movement of our hand sometimes controlling the direction, and often surprising us by what we have
drawn, gives us a sense of having given our ideas voice, expression, or completion. Sometimes meaning can emerge from
what you have created—an understanding of what is happening
in a given situation.

A woman who took a series of stress management classes
from me told me that she often hyperventilates and sometimes even has to be taken to the hospital. However, when this
occurred after having done some art activities in my class, she
quickly got out the new box of crayons she had bought herself
and got involved. By focusing on the colors and expressing herself, she was able to relax and stop hyperventilating.

Someone once said that architecture is frozen music. In that case, I see movement and dance as drawing invisible art in space. Art is also another means of movement. When showing an art piece, I point out the flow of movement on the paper. In a group, if we do movement activities first, we then draw and interpret what we have felt or done. Sometimes we move so as to interpret someone else's art work. Other times, we might draw first and then interpret the drawing by moving either one body part or the whole body, dancing. The following are ideas for movement on paper and in space.

THREE-PART DRAWINGS

This is a process I use when I want to give the group a way to visualize what is taking place in the body and mind after three different kinds of activities. At the very beginning of a session, ask everyone to draw his or her mood. Tell the group that they may draw anything in any way they want to, from abstract to realistic, using crayons and Magic Markers. Do a second drawing after a movement sequence, and a third drawing after a relaxation exercise. Compare and discuss the drawings at the end of the session. With the group in a circle, ask participants to place their drawings in front of them, facing the outside of the circle, with the first drawing on the left, the second drawing in the middle, and the third drawing on the right. When comparing the differences from the first to the third, look for change in colors and how the space is used, the change from realistic to more abstract style, and increases of energy in the second drawings. The energy is often transformed to the center of the page in the third one. For example, they usually can see a calm, quiet quality in their drawings made after the relaxation exercise. These changes are not universal and are not done as art therapy. The purpose is merely to visually see what the body and mind have experienced. Sometimes it is not expressed in the drawings and sometimes it is.

INTERPRETING COLORS

Have a discussion about what a specific color means to each person in the group, and how this color makes him or her feel.

You might start with red and display a few red items, such as a red scarf, red crayons, and red construction paper. Bring in red objects, such as red pipe cleaners, buttons, tissue paper, and colored pictures from magazines. You may want to explore how this color has been used in an advertisement on T.V. or in a movie to evoke feelings.

After discussing feelings about this color, ask for movement that might express the color (Figure 34) and put this movement into a dance. You also may want to ask the participants to do a drawing or collage all in one color, individually or as a group.

DRAW AND MOVE

Another way to initiate a multi-arts project is to start with music. Choose a dramatic piece of music without words and have the group close their eyes, listen, and then do a drawing depicting the images in their imagination or their interpretation of the music. This can be followed by writing a poem about the music.

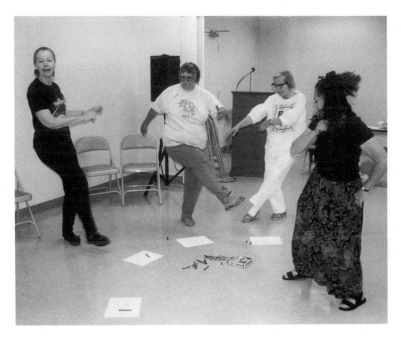

Figure 34. Interpreting colors into movements.

You also can start with a piece of art work and let the group write a poem about what they see, followed by choreographing a dance to express the painting.

INTERPRET MUSIC WITH DRAWING AND DANCE

Have each person lead a recording with a stick or a crayon as a baton playing a chosen piece of music, such as a waltz. Suggest that the rest of the group follow the person conducting with a body part (e.g., lead the orchestra with your head, finger, or elbow). A scarf can be tied to the stick to give the movement more flow or a bannerlike quality.

Then distribute paper and crayons and ask participants to allow the movement of conducting to flow onto the paper, using as many colors as they wish (Figure 35). If it is difficult to move the group to a table, trays can be distributed and the drawings can be done on laps.

When the music has been stopped and everyone is finished, have each member display his or her drawing, while the whole group interprets each drawing with body part and whole-body movement, first without the music and then with the music.

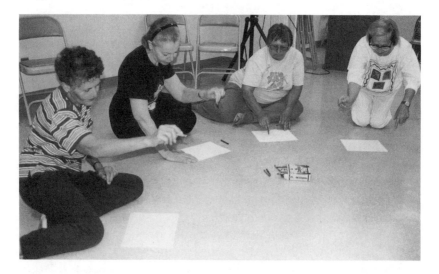

Figure 35. Conducting the music.

Try this with different types of music, some flowing, like the waltz, and some staccato, such as disco. The differences in drawings and movement will range from curved and circular lines (waltz) to sharp, jagged, and angular lines (disco). For some people there will be little change. There will be a variety of interpretations for each piece of music, even though everyone is interpreting the same piece of music.

MURALS AND GROUP DRAWINGS

Individual drawings can be put together to make a group collage. You can start by choosing a subject, and have the group do a mural after discussion. Or, pass one large piece of paper from person to person, having each add to it to make one mural. In addition, a group mural can be done to interpret a group poem. Where possible, tape a large sheet of paper to the wall. A physically fit group can move around each other and draw on different sections of the paper.

Interpreting music with art and movement also can be done as a group mural, with everyone working at once, perhaps moving to other people's drawings. The movement can interpret the mural section by section, or the group can interpret any part of the mural they wish in small groups or all together, standing or in chairs.

As an addition to this activity, each person can look for images in their scribbles and bring them out with Magic Markers or oil pastels. Follow this with sharings and discussion.

STRAW DRAWINGS

This activity can help promote deeper breathing as well as expand the creative imagination. Dilute tempera paint with water, testing to find the right consistency that will flow smoothly but is not too watery. Place about one tablespoon of this mixture on a piece of paper for each person. Have each person take a drinking straw and blow directly onto the paint. (Be sure to warn the group not to suck in, or they will inhale the paint.) The air will blow the paint into designs they can devise.

When these are finished, the process can be extended by using the imagination and creating another picture. Have everyone share their straw drawing and ask what each person sees. Remind them to allow their imaginations to go wild. Then let them add to their drawing with crayons, carrying the composition further in any way that occurs to them. This activity would not be appropriate for confused persons.

ADDITIONAL ART PROJECTS

3-D Body Tracings

Have the group trace body parts on a doubled sheet of butcher block paper, and then cut out and stuff with newspaper, stapling along the way. Body tracings can also be done without stuffing by tracing hands and feet several times, coloring them, and pasting them on another sheet in any way desired, including an overlapping pattern.

String Painting

Have participants dip string in paint and then wiggle the string on paper. The group can experiment with different colors; when the paint is wet, the colors may run or smear, which could also be interesting. After the string painting dries, it can be left as is or shapes can be defined, changed, or turned into a collage with other art supplies.

Textures

Abstract or realistic pictures can be made using squares of waxed paper, foil, plastic, felt, sand, buttons, colored cotton balls, etc.

Rubbings can be done on any surface that is not smooth. For those who can move around the room, or even outside, allow them to be creative and do rubbings from anything they like. Indoors, it could be any signs that are embossed or cut out, grills of heating vents, screening, cork bulletin boards, or sockets. Outdoors, it could be tree trunks, cement pavements, or pebbled paths. Or, you can bring in objects such as leaves, acorns, feathers, sandpaper, and books whose titles can be rubbed.

Art therapist Annette Rosso-Sloan makes the following suggestion. After doing rubbings, discuss what each person sees in his or her own rubbings. Participants can begin by saying, "I see," "I am," "I feel," "I know," etc., about themselves.

Sponge Painting

Using different-shaped sponges and a variety of paint colors, allow the participants to dip each of their sponges into a different color and blot each on a sheet of paper. The walls of an entire room can be painted in this way.

Puppets

Paper plates and even envelopes can be creatively used to make hand puppets. Egg cartons can be cut into three sections and each section can be designed as a "Big Mouth" puppet. After the puppets have been created, you can have them answer the same questions that are suggested for poetry subjects.

Collages

The group can paste tissue paper and torn paper designs on a light-colored poster board or a sheet of paper. Have things cut out, ready to go, and allow each person a choice of what he or she would like to use, without overwhelming participants with too many choices.

PART IV

INTERGENERATIONAL ACTIVITIES AND IDEAS FOR ADAPTING ACTIVITIES FOR OLDER ADULTS WITH SPECIAL NEEDS

Chapter 14

Bridging the Generations Through Movement

[D]espite our differences, we're all alike. Beyond identities and desires there is a common core of self—an essential humanity whose nature is peace and whose expression is thought and whose action is unconditional love. When we identify with that inner core, respecting and honoring it in others as well as ourselves, we experience healing in every area of life.

—Joan Borysenko

We, or our societal structures, often isolate ourselves into categorized groups. These groups can be based on disability, race, or cultural background. In some areas, this segregation of people has changed somewhat. Today there is more mainstreaming of physically, mentally, and emotionally challenged children into regular schools. There also is a growing interest in intergenerational programs, programs that bring together different generations. I was involved with one program that brought teenagers together with older adults for fitness and relaxation, and another that brought preschool children together with older adults for creative dance and exercise. In another program, funded by the District of Columbia Commission on the Arts and Humanities and the National Endowment for the Arts, I trained a group of adults of varied ages and cultural backgrounds to work with older adults in senior centers using movement and related activities.

186 / Intergenerational Activities and Special Needs

It is often difficult to obtain funding for programs. Because there are some funds available for older adults and some for children's programs, it makes sense not only for the benefits that can be derived for both age groups but also for practical purposes to create intergenerational programs. I feel it is important to reach out and include as many participants as possible, and to be aware of the support system in each facility. It is also important to utilize and integrate as much of the facility and the community as possible. Using the activities in this book and a bit of creativity, anyone can design an intergenerational program to fit the specific needs of a facility or school. The remainder of the chapter details one such program.

SHILOH-KENDALL CREATIVE MOVEMENT PROGRAM

In 1988–1989, I carried out an intergenerational creative movement program with older adults with hearing impairment, ages 60–88, from Shiloh Senior Center and children, ages 10–12, from the Kendall Demonstration Middle School at Gallaudet University, the first university in the world for persons with hearing impairments. This program also was made possible through a grant from the District of Columbia Commission on the Arts and Humanities and the National Endowment for the Arts.

The makeup of the group changed slightly over the years. When possible, however, consistent child–adult partners were established. Each set of partners developed a segment of what the group would do together in each dance for the performances. This created bonding but allowed the partners to get to know each other while learning from others.

Bringing children and adults with hearing impairment together was a rewarding experience that stretched us all. In the process of creating and practicing, the children and older adults began to appreciate, respect, and know each other. For many of the children, this was their first interaction with older deaf persons. And, because none of the seniors involved had deaf children or grandchildren, their own interaction with such children was limited. Initially, the question they all asked each other was "Are you deaf?"

When designing the program, I focused only on the intergenerational hearing impairment aspect. I was aware that times had changed greatly for deaf persons. Not only had the older adults learned to accept many more societal limitations while growing up, but there were some communication problems because the older adults used signs for some words that were different from the signs that the children used. These sorts of differences affected the relationships, but also expanded the exposure and experiences of both groups; each learned more about themselves as well as others.

First-Year Program

The first year's performance program consisted of "Nonlocomotor Movements," "Poem Enactments," "Body Breaths," and "A Scarf Dance." First, in pairs, we explored statue poses (Figure 36) of each of the nonlocomotor movements of stretch, bend, twist, shake, strike, push, and pull. For hearing audiences, we taught the signs for each of these words before we started. Each word statue was done three times in three statue freezes, with the participants in constant physical contact with their partners. We invited the audience to join us in the third one by performing it in their seats. The whole group then introduced and explored each of four chosen nonlocomotor words. Each of the children had scripted these words, and performed them in movement at the same time after their introduction. First the children held each word pose for four counts; then they held each word pose for one count, changing the word pose quickly; and then they took four counts to complete each word pose, so that it was done in slow motion. This segment concluded with all on stage connecting to one another to make one statue of the whole group using the word *bend* as the pose influence. We asked for and chose members of the audience to come up and become part of this statue.

Next on the program was an enactment of a poem written by some of the group. Each person recited and signed one line and then performed it in mime with his or her partner, and sometimes with others in the group. The following poem was interpreted:

> When I was a child
>   I played baseball.
> When I grow up
>   I want to become an artist.

When I was a child
  I was always fighting with my
  brothers and sisters.
When I grow up
  I'm gonna dance and perform every year.
When I was a child
  I played jump rope.
When I grow up
  I want to be an author.
When I was a child.
  I played horseshoes.

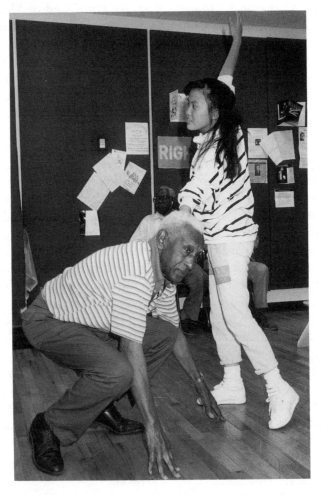

Figure 36.   An intergenerational game of statues.

The third piece in the program, "Body Breaths," again was done with partners facing each other. As one partner breathed in slowly and moved up, the other breathed out and moved down in time with the breath. Each pair explored ways of expanding and contracting the body in time with the breath, which changed from slow to fast. This creative dance also explored the breath energy and movement qualities of sneezing, coughing, and laughing. The program ended with a scarf dance, using scarves as the initiator of movement and ended with everyone throwing the scarves up in the air and then floating to the floor with the scarves.

Taped music was used for all the dances. A large kettle drum whose vibrations could be felt was used to signal changes in the dances. The video and television department at Gallaudet taped parts of the program, which was aired on "Deaf Mosaics" and "Fantastics," and was broadcast on PBS. (Using the media for visibility of your program can help you obtain future funding and volunteers.)

Second-Year Program

During the second year, the program consisted of "Bridges," "Name Rhythms," "Over, Under, Round, and Round," and "Accents." "Bridges" grew out of the concept of a bridge that connects two things. Each person made a bridge statue with his or her body that was held for a few counts. They next did this with a partner, then in groups of three, and continued adding more people until the entire group was making one connecting bridge.

"Name Rhythms" (for a description, see Chapter 4) was extended by having each person design a movement to go with his or her name rhythm. Then each person taught his or her movement rhythm to the whole group, and we developed the dance rhythms into a group pattern and dance.

The third dance, "Over, Under, Round, and Round," grew out of a session held only with the children, on a day when the older adults couldn't make it because of a bus problem. We were exploring the concepts of *over, under,* and *turning* with our bodies. Each child created his or her own individual way to turn or spin, which was then taught to the rest of the class. We did these in a sequence and then found ways to crawl over and under each other when we were in a group formation.

The last dance was "Accents." Using a four-count beat, the dancers divided into four groups. On each of the four counts, one of the groups performed an improvised body movement so that each group accented a different count. One group moved on the count of one, another on the count of two, and so on. Before performing this piece, we explained the process to the audience and divided them in four sections so they could join in by first clapping it out with us, then doing a movement in their seats, and finally joining the performers who were doing the dance on stage by dancing in their seats. All of these pieces were done to either music or a drum beat.

Program Benefits

Because I wanted to reach as many people as possible with this program, teacher workshops were offered. I was able to do an improvisation workshop with the Gallaudet University Dance Company, where I presented movement as music and rhythm ideas. During the second year, three students from the music department at Gallaudet developed compositions that were used for the final performances.

As far as I know, it was unique to bring together generations of hearing persons and persons with hearing impairment of all races and educational and economic backgrounds and, through dance and the art of creation, help them find a common ground or stage. The special joys of the program included the participants' growing understanding and appreciation of dance and the art of performing before varied audiences. Other accomplishments included the increased pride of the participants, the growing relationships between the children and the older adults, and sharing parts of themselves throughout the program. After the program, the principal of the Kendall Middle School said, "The many threads that bind human hearts and minds can be woven beautifully through the art of creative expressions."

Chapter 15

Special Activities for Participants Who Are Very Frail or Have Cognitive Impairments

Unfortunately, too many people think that creativity is something mysterious that only belongs to certain people, whereas everyone has access to it.

—John Cage

Sometimes, in a multipurpose adult senior center a group is mixed in physical and mental ability. Adult day care centers usually have members with a variety of functional abilities. In long-term care facilities, you may be able to separate participants with cognitive impairment into one small group. As a facilitator, you must be very creative as well as sensitive to the individual needs of each participant. In that case, it is up to you to try many different activities to see what will motivate each person to respond. Without being there with you, it is difficult for me to say what will or will not work for you; I can only make suggestions. Ultimately, *you* will have to choose. Throughout this book there are activities that will be appropriate for you no matter what group or individual you are serving.

In working with very frail or low-functioning people, you might more readily burn out if you are attached to the outcome of your service. I remember one of the first times I was in a very large and depressing long-term care facility. The staff were apathetic, the place smelled of urine, the walls were bare of color or art, and most of the residents in the lounge where I was to do the class were either sleeping in their chairs or staring into space. My initial response was disgust. I had an agenda, a program I had planned and expected to get responses from. At first, nothing happened. Finally, I began to look into the eyes of first one individual and then another as I spoke to them. I began to really see and relate to each person, letting go of how he or she would respond to the activity, letting go of who was leading and who following. Instead of being attached to my role and the outcome, I opened my heart and was there, in the moment, human being to human being with love. By the time I left, those who were asleep had awakened, most had responded to me in some way, some asked when I would be back, and I no longer was aware of the smell of urine.

In the book, *How Can I Help? Stories and Reflections on Service,* by Ram Dass and Paul Gorman (1987), the authors state,

> It's not always our efforts that burn us out; it's where the mind is standing in relation to them. The problem is not the work itself but the degree of our identification with it....Taking our initiative personally means taking their consequences personally, too. All these conditions seem inevitably to lead to frustration, fatigue, and burnout....when we break through and meet in spirit behind our separateness, we experience profound moments of companionship. These, in turn, give us access to deeper and deeper levels of generosity and loving kindness. True compassion arises out of unity...."To forget the Self is to be enlightened by all things"....Our service, then, is less a function of personal motive and more an expression of spontaneous, appropriate caring. (pp.197–216)

Caring and compassion are more important than the activities, but if you care, and have some knowledge and creativity, you will find a way to interest and influence participation of some kind.

ACTIVITIES FOR FRAIL PERSONS

Body Part Articulation and Passive/Active

For an individual who must remain in bed, you might want to gently move the head and limbs in many directions, lifting and circling where and when you can and *never, never* forcing. As mentioned in the Passive/Active activity (see Chapter 6), you could suggest the image of being as loose as a rag doll and then ask if the person can hold the arm or leg in the position you placed it in for a moment or more. You may either release the limb and let it fall, if appropriate, or place it back on the bed. This activity provides the opportunity for caring touch as well as articulated movement of body parts.

Mirroring

If possible, try to influence self-motivated movement, using either props or ideas suggested in this book. Mirroring (see Chapter 6) also may initiate some participation, depending on the energy and cognitive ability of the person. Try to take turns, first letting him or her lead with a movement or gesture. Then you lead, keeping in mind the strength and ability of this person.

Touch, Hit, or Kick

Using balloons or other objects tied to the bed, ceiling, or wall by a string, thread, or colorful ribbon, suggest that a person who must remain in bed reach for, touch, hit, or kick the objects. You might even give the suggestions in a sequential order for memory enhancement, if appropriate.

ACTIVITIES FOR PERSONS
WITH COGNITIVE IMPAIRMENT

A Parachute Scarf

A very large, lightweight (silklike), colorful scarf held by one person at each corner can be lifted up and down, in unison. Balloons can be added in the center (Figure 37). This also works well with a parachute. A sheet or a lightweight tablecloth

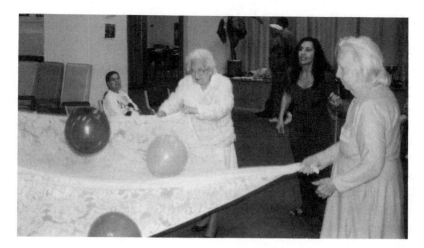

Figure 37.   Participants use a table cloth to toss and catch balloons.

could also be used if available. For ambulatory participants, one person can try to move under the scarf while it is lifted up and get out before it is brought down. Or, if it is brought down on the person (with permission), he or she can make shapes, pushing one or more body parts against the scarf or parachute.

Puppets

Felt body parts with Velcro on their backs can be cut out for participants to place in the proper positions on a large puppet or felt cutout of a person for body part awareness.

I have great success with hand puppets. Participants can communicate with each other verbally or nonverbally, by just having the puppets move. By doing this, they are also flexing their fingers and hands, as well as being motivated to participate.

Doors–Floors

In a workshop I took with Melanie Chavin, author of *The Lost Cord*, she made the following suggestions for persons who tend to drift or pace around or wander from the room:

1.   Move the door handle to an unexpected place, such as very low and close to the floor, or higher than usual.
2.   Invite an art class from a senior center to paint a design or scene on the door and around the door handle so that

the handle becomes part of the design or scene and is disguised.

3.   Have some hands-on activities set up along the walls and around the room so that pacers and drifters can participate as they go by.

Over, Under, In, and Out

For those who are physically able, and are not frightened by confined spaces, large cardboard boxes can be used to climb in and out of. Hula hoops placed on the floor can be used for the same purpose. Crawling under and over objects and stepping in and out of objects help reinforce these concepts, as well as utilize large muscle groups.

Elastic

Large pieces of elastic and inner tubes can be used for pulling and stretching as exercise for the arms. The facilitator may want to hold the other end of a piece of elastic. A textured thick rope can be used for a rope tug. The elastic with bells (see Chapter 5) would be appropriate for some as well.

Senses

When using textures (see Chapter 9), you can add colored tissue paper to crumple and listen to, and colored cellophane to wrap very loosely around the head for a sensory experience, if appropriate. Again, I remind you to be sensitive to each person's fears.

Finger Paints and Clay

For finger painting, use marshmallow cream, vanilla pudding, or whipped cream with food coloring, so there will be no danger if they are placed in the mouth.

Here is a recipe for edible Play-Doh, which can be used in place of clay:

1/2 cup of peanut butter
1/4 cup of honey
1 cup powdered milk

In a bowl, mix the peanut butter, honey, and 1/2 cup of the powdered milk with your hands. Keep adding the rest of the

powdered milk until the dough feels soft and not sticky.
(Check on dietary restrictions for individuals who may use
these ingredients.)

RESOURCE IDEAS

Recently, I was taken on a tour of a nursing home. In the wing
for residents with dementia and Alzheimer's disease, I was
shown one room that appalled me. The room was devoid of
stimulation, except for a mural on the wall. There was no staff
person, no activity, just a room filled with people sitting at an
oblong table or along the walls, some just staring into space
and others talking but making no sense or contact with anyone. This was very surreal. When we left, I asked, somewhat
sarcastically, "Is that supposed to be social interaction?!!" My
guide explained that the center was understaffed and that, as
the activity director, she would rather have them in a room
together than all alone in their rooms.

I believe this situation is a problem in many places. How
can we address this? Perhaps by using students at nearby col-
leges who are studying any of the arts, dance, therapy, recreation, and/or gerontology. They could be offered the possibility
of doing a project or just volunteering some time. Community
religious organizations and well elderly persons also could be
resources. Intergenerational programming would be of great
value in facilities such as these. Volunteers could easily be
trained to do some activities with the residents or at least to
visit with them, if only to make some human contact for short
periods of time.

PART V

PUTTING IT ALL TOGETHER

Chapter 16

Sample Classes
and Workshops

Nobody grows old by merely living a number of years. People grow old only by deserting their ideals. Years may wrinkle the skin but to give up interest wrinkles the soul.
                                            —General Douglas MacArthur

SAMPLE CLASSES

This book includes a wide range of activities that can be put together in many different ways to make up a class. Any number of these pieces will make a whole no matter how they are ordered. Class leaders can select something from each of the chapters, mixing and matching as many activities as desired. Each leader must decide what will work best for him or her and for the participants of each particular class.

The types of activities, and the specific activities within these types, that are chosen will depend on several factors: the time frame, the leader's goals, the group being served, and the leader's professional/personal background. For example, a class may be led by an activities professional, a recreational or expressive arts therapist, an occupational or physical therapist, a fitness or exercise professional, a nutritionist, a nurse, a nursing assistant, a companion, or a home health care aide. A class may consist of:

- Very fit, younger older adults who want to be very active and challenged physically and mentally
- Very frail older adults in a long-term care facility who are physically weak but mentally alert

- A group who have dementia and are cognitively impaired
- A mixed group of persons, including those who are fit, those who are frail, and those who have cognitive impairment
- An intergenerational group who may want to develop a performance or presentation

The following examples of classes may guide and help group leaders with plans of their own. These are only samples that can be adjusted to meet specific needs and time frames. By no means are these suggested samples to be accepted, or used, as finalized, inflexible formats; they are *just* an illustration of possibilities. Brainstorming and sharing with other professionals in one's field is another way to add life to such programs.

Fitness Classes

A Frail but Alert Group Frail but alert persons may live in a long-term care facility or a retirement facility with independent living and partial care. A typical class for such individuals could include the following activities:

- Introductions with a musical instrument (Chapter 1)
- A breath awareness activity (Chapter 1)
- Chair exercises (any number and in any order that seems appropriate for the group) (Chapter 7)
- One creative activity using a prop (Chapter 5), such as scarves, or a dance idea (Chapter 4), such as the Charleston or the bunny hop done in a sitting position
- An uplifting last activity before the closing, such as a group poem (Chapter 12) or reading some uplifting quotes
- A group closure (described later in this chapter) and hugs

A Fit and Active Group Fit and active persons may participate in activities at senior centers or recreation centers, in adult evening classes, or in elderhostel programs. A typical class for such individuals could include the following activities:

- Introductions using name with movement (Chapter 4)
- Chair, mat, and standing exercises (Chapter 7), which are appropriate for this group
- A creative activity or two, such as nonlocomotor movements, scripts, and statues (Chapter 3) and "Open/Close" or "Fill-Ins" (Chapter 6)
- A relaxation or imagery exercise and "Hands-On" (Chapter 8).
- A group closure and hugs

"More than Movement" Classes

A Group with Mixed Physical and Cognitive Abilities Such individuals may be found in some senior centers, nutrition centers, and multipurpose centers. A typical class for these individuals could include the following activities:

- Introductions with rhythm sounds and group echoes using a musical instrument (Chapter 1)
- A deep breathing awareness exercise (Chapter 1), followed by the deep breathing exercise at the beginning of Chapter 7
- Body part warm-ups and dances (Chapter 4)
- "Category Dances" (Chapter 4)
- Moving with balloons (Chapter 5)
- Chinese jump ropes (Chapter 5)
- "Drum Up Energy" (Chapter 6)
- "Draw and Move" or interpreting music with drawing and dance (Chapter 13)
- "Remembering and Sharing" (Chapter 10); could be developed into a poem or story and interpreted in pantomime
- Group closure and hugs

A Group with Cognitive Impairment Persons with cognitive impairment may live in a long-term care facility, in an adult day care center, or at home. Props, rhythm, and music usually work best to stimulate those individuals with dementia. For persons with cognitive impairment, smaller groups are best for more individualized attention, and shorter sessions are probably more effective. A typical class for these individuals could include the following activities:

- Introductions and welcome with a musical instrument (Chapter 1)
- One or more of the deep breathing and breath awareness activities in Chapter 1
- Any of the activities from Chapter 15 (e.g., body part articulation; touch, hit, or kick; a parachute scarf; sensory stimulation; finger paints and clay)
- One or more of the movement motivators and props from Chapter 5 (e.g., bells on ankles and wrists, soft dolls, "Kick the Cookie Can")
- Exercises exploring senses (Chapter 9)

- Sing-alongs (Chapter 2); the class leader must be prepared to vary, simplify, or eliminate the structured movement
- A closure of hugs

Sample Classes for Specific Service Providers

The following suggestions for class content are grouped according to the needs of *specific service providers*. I recommend that each class begin with an appropriate introduction from Chapter 1. Also, when suitable, try to include at least one breathing awareness activity; one body part warm-up; one or more creative and fun activities; a mixture of arts, such as music, poetry, art, and dance; an uplifting activity; and a closure with hugs.

Occupational Therapists   Occupational therapists may wish to use the pantomime activities, such as category dances, and some of the elements of movement from Chapter 3, as well as mirroring (Chapter 6).

Physical Therapists   Physical therapists may want to use activities that will motivate their clients to move the specific body parts in need of therapy while having fun, so that they can then move the clients into the more specific or difficult physical therapy exercises. Some of the activities in this book may even offer ideas on how to vary standard physical therapy exercises to make them more creative, interesting, and fun. The movement motivators and props in Chapter 5 are fun ways to extend movement without the feeling of hard work. The imagery of the "Freedom Dance" in Chapter 8 may enhance the actual movement. Using a self-expressive art, such as those in Chapters 12 and 13, can help clients to regain self-esteem and release pent-up emotions. "Emotion/Motion" (Chapter 4) can also help clients to express emotions nonverbally or verbally.

Expressive Arts Therapists   Expressive arts therapists may wish to select activities from arts other than their particular specialties (e.g., dance therapists may choose art activities from Chapter 13), or they may integrate more than one art form, as suggested in the haiku multi-art process in Chapter 12. The "Emotion/Motion" and "Hand Dance" exercises in Chapter 4 may be appropriate to reach deeply blocked emotions in persons with mental illness. For example the "Open/Close," "Wide/Narrow," "Expand/Contract," "Grow/ Shrink," and

"Unfold/Fold" activities in Chapter 6 can help to expand movement vocabulary which can be translated into expression of the personality. For instance, reaching further out with the body can be related to reaching further out verbally. If there is fear of reaching out with the body, a discussion of the fear of reaching out in general can follow. Many of the creative activities described in this book may stimulate changes in routine activities. Modifying a tried and true activity can add zest and new life to it.

Nurses and Nursing Assistants Any nurses and nursing assistants who have time to be with their patients for more than medical care may want to enhance their caring touch with suggestions from the section on the importance of touch in Chapter 8. Some creative activities, such as those on the senses in Chapter 9, can be used by bringing an object with a different texture each time rounds are made. A conversation can be started with the patient about the texture: its feel, its look, or the memories it stimulates. There are additional ideas for working with textures in Chapter 13. Other related activities are sensory stimulation and puppets (Chapter 15); a puppet can be carried along on rounds. The exercises on imagery in Chapter 8 may also be of benefit.

Family Caregivers and Home Health Care Aides Home health care aides may want to draw on activities that will awaken, occupy, and interest their clients, and that give the opportunity to share and listen. Sing-alongs and matching movement to rhythm (Chapter 2) and exploring the elements of movement (Chapter 3) would be beneficial if appropriate in a given situation. Story dances, as described in Chapter 4, and perception expanders (Chapter 9), as well as "This Is Your Life" (Chapter 10), may also be useful.

Intergenerational Classes

Intergenerational programs can utilize almost all the activities in this book depending on the ages of the children and the abilities of the older adults, as well as the focus of the program. Whenever possible, one older adult should be paired with one child for bonding a closer, more personal relationship. If preschool or kindergarten children are grouped together with physically able older adults for creative movement classes, the focus can be on relating movement and arts to the cognitive concepts of shape, space, time, and force, as in Chapter 3, or "Open/Close" and the like, as in Chapter 6. Any of the movement motivators and props in Chapter 5 would also be appropriate with this age group. With an older group of children, "Music, Math, and Movement," from Chapter 2, and "Laban Effort/Shape," from Chapter 3, might be more challenging. If the focus of the group is to create a performance or an informal presentation, the format described in Chapter 14 can be used.

SHARING SUCCESSFUL CLASS METHODS

Class leaders who are feeling comfortable with the methods in this book, have been utilizing them for a period of time, and have found them successful may want to share them with fellow staff or members of an organization to which they belong. The following are the goals, objectives, and contents of two training workshops I give.

Workshop on Motivating
Movement, Having Fun, and Reducing Stress

Goal: To learn how to create an activity program, or session, for the whole person using novel and innovative ideas.

Objectives:

1. Motivate movement, fun, and creativity
2. Increase joint and body part articulation, flexibility, and balance
3. Utilize the arts and positive thought to uplift the whole person
4. Enhance awareness and perceptual skills and reawaken the senses
5. Acquire techniques for memory reinforcement and communication skills to develop easier social interactions
6. Stimulate greater cognizance of breathing and body movements to reduce stress

Contents:

• Introduction and name reinforcements with a musical instrument
• Breathing and stretching, adding use of voice and diaphragm; use of pinwheels, bubbles, and candles as initiators of activities

- Body part warm-ups/joint articulation/range-of-motion concepts
  –Nonlocomotor movements (bend, stretch, twist, shake, etc.): explore each with whole body or body part; script together as a dance; make individual and group statues
  –Category dances: sports, party, farming, housework, name with a movement, or other categories that include movement
- Taking care of the caregiver (Beating Burnout): stress reduction and relaxation techniques, imagery, cognitive distortions, and thought stopping
- Techniques for creating poetry and sharing oral histories to enhance memory, self-expression, communication, and social interactions in order to feel better about the whole self
- Methods for focusing on the positive
- Using textures to awaken the senses
- Moving in your mind's eye: imagery set to music and creative visualization followed by drawing or describing what was visualized
- Drumming up energy: playing imaginary drums with different body parts
- Using props, songs, and ideas to motivate and stimulate participation: scarves and streamers, cookie can, bean bags as weights, lightweight dolls, puppets, squeeze toys, rainbow glasses, worry dolls, and the like; ways to create activities with these
- Stimulating social interaction through movement fun: fill-in's, passive/active, and tissue introductions
- Brainstorming in groups

Workshop on Taking Care of the Caregiver

Goal: To develop tools for living your joy, stress alleviation, and giving yourself permission to love yourself and therefore others.

Objectives:

1. Learn tools for balancing the body, mind, and spirit.
2. Learn practical and creative stress reduction activities, including moving with fun; deep breathing and relaxation techniques; imagery; journal writing; creative self-expression through dancing, art, poetry, and drumming.

3. Develop techniques of thought stopping, refuting irrational ideas, determining the meaning and threats of your stressors, and looking at cognitive distortions.
4. Find ways to uplift the spirit.

Contents:

- Playful introductions
- Breathing and stretching
- Body part warm-ups: creative ways to loosen muscles and joints (exercising without exercise)
- Creative self-expression: using all the arts
- Relaxation techniques: quieting the mind through deep breathing and concentration
- Cognitive distortions: how we think and the effects of our thoughts
- Thought stopping and reframing
- Imagery and visualization
- Massage techniques to release tense muscles
- Discussion and questions

CLOSURE: WAYS OF ENDING A CLASS

At the end of a recent presentation I did for senior citizens at a retirement facility, one of the participants came up to me and said, "I kept looking at my watch because I didn't want the class to end." This touched me and I realized that, when I am teaching, I am also having such a good time that the time flies by. However, every class must come to an end, and a formal closure can make this more meaningful.

I end all of my classes where possible with a hand-holding circle, including those who have to remain in their chairs (we arrange our circle to include these chairs, unless it is too difficult, time consuming, or inappropriate). I ask all the participants to close their eyes. Then I say, "Take a deep breath all the way to your toes, filling your body with all the goodness in the world and, when you breathe out, breathe out all the garbage you no longer need—all the problems, pains, worries, fears, and negative thoughts. Breathe in all the love in the world. Open your hearts and fill your bodies with light and love. Then breathe out and share this love with everyone in this room, feeling it pass from hand to hand, round and round the circle. Now breathe in all the love in the entire universe and share it with the whole world." I complete this by saying, "Thank you for sharing this time with me." Some people may feel uneasy or embarrassed saying this, but I find that all my groups enjoy this tremendously, including those participating in staff training.

Sometimes I suggest that everyone imagine a person they know, who needs healing, is in the center of our circle. I ask all of them to send their love and prayers to the center of the circle. I also may ask everyone to open their eyes and make loving eye contact with each person in the circle.

I always end with everyone giving each other hugs. For immobile or frail people, I go to each and share a hug. When I hug, I try to hug honestly, with warmth, feeling love from my heart. I tell everyone I am a collector of hugs. If someone says, "I only have one arm to hug you with," I tell him or her, "All the love you have to share can come through one arm." Then I thank each person for being present and say, "I'll see you next class!"

With the very frail I go to each, ask if they have a hug for me, then take their hands, look into their eyes, and say, "Thank you for being here," and if appropriate I say, "I'll see you next class" (I state the day), and then I say, "God Bless You."

References

American Association of Retired Persons. (1984). *Truth about aging: Guidelines for accurate communications.* Washington, DC: Author.

Baldwin, C. (1991). *Life's companion: Journal writing as a spiritual quest.* New York: Bantam.

Bry, A. (1979). *Visualization directing.* New York: Harper & Row.

Buscaglia, L. (1982). *Living, loving, & learning.* Thorofare, NJ: SLACK, Inc.

Chavin, M. (1991). *The lost cord: Reaching the person with dementia through the power of music.* Mt. Airy, MD: Elder Song Publication.

Cousins, N. (1979). *Anatomy of an illness as perceived by the patient.* New York: Bantam.

Cousins, N. (1992). Norman Cousins. In P. Berman & C. Goldman (Eds.), *The ageless spirit* (pp. 43–49). New York: Ballantine Books.

Dass, R., & Gorman, P. (1987). *How can I help? Stories and reflections on service.* New York: Alfred A. Knopf.

Elkin, A. (1989, August). 6 tranquilizers and how to use them: Time tested techniques to calm you down fast. *Prevention Magazine,* 41–46.

Feil, N. (1993). *The validation breakthrough: Simple techniques for communicating with people with "Alzheimer's-type dementia."* Baltimore: Health Professions Press.

Fiatarone, M.A., O'Neil, E.F., Doyle-Ryan, N., Clements, K.M., Solareo, G.R., Nelson, M.E., Roberts, S.B., Kehayia, J.J., Lipsitz, L.A., & Evans, W.J. (1994). Exercise training and nutritional supplements for physical frailty in very elderly people. *New England Journal of Medicine, 330*(25), 1769–1775.

Gawain, S. (1983). *Creative visualization.* New York: Bantam.

Goleman, D. (1988, February 2). The experience of touch: Research points to a critical role. *New York Times,* p. C1.

Jampolsky, G. (1984). *Teach only love.* New York: Bantam.

Lowen, A. (1976). *Bioenergetics.* New York: Penguin Books.

Maas, M.S., & Kuypers, J.A. (1974). *From 30 to 70: A forty-year longitudinal study of adult life styles and personality.* San Francisco: Jossey-Bass.

Manheimer, R. (1986). Creative arts: A threshold to renewed life. *Perspectives on Aging.*

Moen, L. (1992). *Guided imagery* (Vol. II). Naples, FL: United States Publishing.

Montague, A. (1971). *Touching: The human significance of the skin.* New York: Columbia University Press.

Roman, S. (1986). *Living with joy: Keys to personal power and spiritual transformation.* Tiburon, CA: H.J. Kramer, Inc.

Roth, G. (1989). *Maps to ecstasy: teaching of an urban shamon.* Novato, CA: Nataraj Publishers.

Rozman, D. (1975). *Meditating with children: New age meditations for children. the art of concentrating and centering.* Boulder Creek, CA: Planetary Publications.

Shorr, J. (1977). *Go see the movie in your head.* Santa Barbara, CA: Ross-Erikson.

Siegel, B. (1986). *Love, medicine, and miracles.* New York: Harper & Row.

Simonton, O.C., Simonton, S.M., & Creighton, J. (1978). *Getting well again: A step-by-step self-help guide to overcoming cancer for patients and their families.* New York: J.P. Tarcher.

Voirst, J. (1989). *Forever 50 and other negotiations.* Taft, TX: S.S. Trade.

Williams, M. (1983). *The velveteen rabbit.* New York: Alfred A. Knopf.

Appendix A

Recommended Music

RECOMMENDED ALBUMS

Alden, Bonnie. *Charleston.* Roulette.
The Alonim Singers. *Wonderful Songs of Israel.* Barclay Recording.
Ave Maria. *Gregorian Chants.* St. Cecilia's Abbey.
Bee Gees. *Bee Gees Greatest.* RSO Records.
Cirque du Soleil. *Cirque du Soleil.* RCA Victor.
Colonel Bogey. *The Great Military Marches.* CBS Records.
The Commitments. *California.* MCA Records.
Crystal Chimes. *In the Enchanted Crystal Forest in Ojai, California.* Inner Circle Records.
Environments. *Slow Ocean.* Syntonic Research, Inc.
Enya. *Shepard Moons.* Reprise.
Enya. *Watermark.* Reprise.
Gabrielle Roth and the Mirrors. *Initiation.* Raven Recording.
Gabrielle Roth and the Mirrors. *Ritual.* Raven Recording.
Gabrielle Roth and the Mirrors. *Waves.* Raven Recording.
Hart, Mickey. *Planet Drum.* Rykodisc, USA.
Horn, Paul. *Inside the Taj Mahal II.* Vancouver Island Productions.
Japanese Koto Orchestra. Lyrichord Discs.
Kano. *Runes by Kano.* Spirit Music.
Kitaro. *Silk Road Suite.* Kuckuck Records.
The Klezmer Conservatory Band. *Klez!* Vanguard Recording Society.
Krupa, Gene. *Drum Boogie.* Columbia Records.
Mantovani. *Strauss Waltzes.* Ffrr.
Margouleff, Robert, & Cecil, Malcolm. *Tonto's Expanding Head Band.* Mediasound Studios.
McFerrin, Bobby. *Simple Pleasures.* Capital Records.
Memphis Slim. *Rock Me Baby.* Black Lion Recording.
Miyata, Koltociro. *Shakohachi—The Japanese Flute.* Elektranonesuch.
Milhaud, Bartok, & Chavez. *Percussion.* Capital Records.

Morton, Jelly Roll. *Plays Jelly Roll.* Olympic Records.
Music for Zen Meditation. Record Industry Association of America.
The Music of Upper and Lower Egypt. Rykodisc, USA.
3 Mustaphas #3. Shanchie.
Olatunji, Babatunde. *Drums of Passion.* Columbia Records.
Perlman, Itzhak, & Previn, Andre. *The Easy Winners.* Angel CD.
Phaedra. *Tangerine Dreams.* Virgin Records.
Rodgers, Richard. *Sound of Music.* Rodgers and Hammerstein Recordings.
Rowland, Mike. *The Fairy Ring.* Narada Distributing.
Spirit Drummers. *Magic.* Primal Productions.
Strauss, Johann, & Strauss, Josef. *Kaiserwalzer Emperor Waltz: Waltzes and Polkas.* Deutsche Grammophon.
Talking Heads. *Speaking in Tongues.* Sire.
Talking Heads. *Stop Making Sense.* Sire.
Thundering Rainstorm. *Nashville.* Silver Bells Music.
Tosh, Peter. *The Toughest.* Capital/EMI.
Varese, Edgar. *Deserts.* Attacca.
Victory Baptist Choir. Sunday Meeting.
Vivaldi, Antonio. *The Four Seasons: Three Concertos From L'estro Armonica.* Polygram Records.
White Pavillion. *Songs with Zuleikha and Friends.* Zuleikha.
Winston, George. *Autumn.* Windham Hill Records.
Winston, George. *December.* Windham Hill Records.
Winston, George. *Winter into Spring.* Windham Hill Records.
Withers, Bill. *Making Friends (The Best You Can).* Still Bill Productions.
Wolff, Henry, & Hennings, Nancy. *Tibetan Bells II.* Celestial Harmonies.

ADDITIONAL RESOURCES

Bi-Folkal Productions, 809 Williamson Street, Madison, Wisconsin 53703. Music, sing-along tapes, and large-print songbooks accompany each of the Bi-Folkal kits. Books may be purchased or borrowed from your local library.
Metro Goldwyn Memories, 5425 West Addison, Chicago, Illinois 60641. Nostalgic recordings, tapes, photos, books, etc. Catalogs are available.
National Association for Music Therapy, Inc., 505 Eleventh Street, S.E., Washington, D.C. 20003. The *Journal of Music* is available for an annual fee.
Reader's Digest Association, Inc., Pleasantville, New York 10570. Reader's Digest offers songbooks such as *Family Songbook, Popular Songs That Will Live Forever, Treasury of Best-Loved*

Songs, Country and Western Songbook, and *Unforgettable Music Memories.*

Recordings for Recovery, Michael Hoy, 413 Cherry, Midland, Michigan 48640. This is a service of taped musical programs available to persons who are institutionalized, homebound, or otherwise limited. For a small annual fee, subscribers are sent a listing of available tapes that they may borrow. This service is handled through the mail, much like Talking Books program.

Appendix B

Suggested Readings

Adler, R.F., & Fisher, P.P. (1984). Myself...through music, movement and art. *The Arts in Psychotherapy, 11*, 203–208.

Albrecht, K. (1979). *Stress and the manager.* Englewood Cliffs, NJ: Prentice Hall.

Alexander, J., and the Calyx Editorial Collective. (Eds.). (1986). *Women and aging: An anthology by women.* Corvallis, OR: Calyx Books.

American Association of Retired Persons. (1984). *Truth about aging: Guidelines for accurate communications.* Washington, DC: Author.

Baldwin, C. (1991). *Life's companion: Journal writing as a spiritual quest.* New York: Bantam.

Bartlett, J., & Snelus, P. (1980). Lifespan memory for popular songs. *American Journal of Psychology, 93*, 551–560.

Batcheller, J., & Monsour, S. (1972). *Music in recreation and leisure.* Dubuque, IA: William C. Brown.

Beal, R.K., & Berryman-Miller, S. (1988). *Focus on dance XI: Dance for the older adult.* Reston, VA: American Alliance for Health, Physical Education, Recreation & Dance.

Berman, P., & Goldman, C. (1992). *The ageless spirit.* New York: Ballantine Books.

Bonny, H. (1990). *Music and your mind.* Barrytown, NY: Station Hill Press.

Borysenko, J. (1987). *Minding the body, mending the mind.* Reading, MA: Addison-Wesley.

Bright, R. (1981). *Music in geriatric care and practical planning in music therapy for the aged.* New York: Musicgraphs.

Bright, R. (1988). *Music therapy and the dementias.* St. Louis, MO: MMB Music, Inc.

Brooks, C.V.W. (1974). *Sensory awareness: Rediscovery of experiencing through the workshops and classes of Charlotte Selver.* New York: Viking Press.

Bry, A. (1979). *Visualization directing.* New York: Harper & Row.

Burns, D. (1980). *Feeling good: The new mood therapy.* New York: Signet.

Buscaglia, L. (1982). *Living, loving, & learning.* Thorofare, NJ: SLACK, Inc.

Caplow-Lindner, E., Harpaz, L., & Samberg, S. (1979). *Therapeutic dance-movement: Expressive activities for older adults.* New York: Human Sciences Press.

Clair, A., & Bernstein, B. (1990). A comparison of singing, vibrotactile and nonvibrotactile instrumental playing responses in severely regressed persons with dementia of the Alzheimer's type. *Journal of Music Therapy, 27,* 119–125.

Colgrove, M., Bloomfield, H., & McWilliams, P. (1976). *How to survive the loss of a love.* New York: Bantam.

Comfort, A. (1976). *Say yes to old age.* New York: Crown Publishers, Inc.

Corbin, D., & Metal-Corbin, J. (1990). *Reach for it!: A handbook of health, exercise and dance activities for older adults* (2nd ed.). Dubuque, IA: Eddie Bowers Publishing, Inc.

Cousins, N. (1979). *Anatomy of an illness as perceived by the patient.* New York: W.W. Norton & Company.

Covey, S. (1989). *The seven habits of highly effective people.* New York: Simon & Schuster.

Dass, R., & Gorman, P. (1987). *How can I help? Stories and reflections on service.* New York: Alfred A. Knopf.

Davis, F. (1971). *Inside intuition.* New York: Signet.

Davis, M., Eshelman, E., & McKay, M. (1982). *The relaxation & stress reduction workbook.* Oakland, CA: New Harbinger Publishing.

Dell, C. (1970). *A primer for movement description using effort shape and supplementary concepts* (2nd rev. ed.). New York: Dance Notation Bureau, Inc.

Douglass, D. (1987). *Accent on rhythm: Music activities for the aged* (3rd rev. ed.). St. Louis, MO: MMB Music, Inc.

Fast, J. (1970). *Body language.* New York: M. Evans & Co., Inc.

Fisher, P.P. (1990, December). Fitness for fun and relaxation. *Greater Washington Senior Beacon,* p. 4.

Fisher, P.P. (1993, March). Controlling your stress. *Diabetes Forecast,* p. 46–47.

Freysinger, V.J., Alessio, H., & Mehdizadeh, S. (1993). Reexamining the morale–physical health–activity relationship: A longitudinal study of time changes and gender differences. *Activities, Adaptation and Aging, 17*(4), 25–41.

Friedman, M.F., & Rosenman, R.H. (1974). *Type A behavior and your heart.* New York: Alfred A. Knopf.

Functional fitness assessment for adults over 60 years. (1990). Reston, VA: American Alliance for Health, Physical Education, Recreation & Dance.

Garnet, E. (1992). *Focus on dance VII: Dance therapy.* Reston, VA: American Alliance for Health, Physical Education, Recreation & Dance.

Gaston, E. (1968). *Music in therapy.* New York: Macmillan.

Gawain, S. (1983). *Creative visualization.* New York: Bantam Books.

Gershon, D., & Straub, G. (1989). *Empowerment: The art of creating your life as you want it.* New York: Delacorte.

Gibbons, A.C. (1977). Popular music preferences of elderly persons. *Journal of Music Therapy, 14,* 180–189.

Gibbons, A.C. (1990). A review of literature for music development/ education and music therapy with the elderly. *Music Therapy Perspectives, 5,* 33–40.

Gillette, P.A. (1993). Senior women's fitness project: A pilot study. *Journal of Women and Aging, 5*(2), 49–66.

Goldberg, P. (1979). *Executive health.* New York: McGraw-Hill.

Goleman, D. (1988, February 2). The experience of touch: Research points to a critical role. *New York Times,* p. C1.

Greenwald, M.A., & Salzberg, R.S. (1979). Vocal range assessment of geriatric clients. *Journal of Music Therapy, 16,* 172–179.

Haber, E.A., & Short-DeGraff, M.A. (1990). Intergenerational programming for an increasingly age-segregated society. *Activities, Adaptation and Aging, 14*(3), 35–49.

Hawkins, A.H. (1991). *Moving from within: A new method for dance making.* Reston, VA: American Alliance for Health, Physical Education, Recreation & Dance.

Helm, J. (1985). *Can you grab a star? Dance/creative arts with older adults: A source book.* New York: Human Sciences Press.

Hirsch, S. (1990). Dance therapy in the service of dementia. *American Journal of Alzheimer's Care and Related Disorders and Research, 5*(4), 26–30.

Hopkins, D.R., et al. (1990). Effect of low-impact aerobic dance on the functional fitness of elderly women. *Gerontologist, 30,* 189–192.

Humor power: How to get it, give it, and gain. New York: Doubleday.

Jaffe, D.T., & Scott, C.D. (1984). *From burnout to balance: A workbook for peak performance and self-renewal.* New York: McGraw-Hill.

Javna, J. (1985). *The TV theme song sing-along song book* (Vol. 2). New York: St. Martin's Press.

Kabat, Z.J. (1990). *Full catastrophe living.* New York: Delacorte.

Karras, B. (1985). *Down memory lane: Topics and ideas for reminiscence groups.* Mt. Airy, MD: Eldersong Publications, Inc.

Katsch, S., & Merle-Fishman, C. (1987). *The music within you.* New York: Simon & Schuster.

Klien, A. (1989). *The healing power of humor.* Los Angeles, CA: Jeremy P. Tarcher, Inc.

Koch, K. (1977). *I never told anybody: Teaching poetry writing in a nursing home.* New York: Vintage Books.

Kriegel, R., & Kriegel, M.H. (1985). *The C zone: Peak performance under pressure.* New York: Fawcett.

Kubler-Ross, E. (1970). *On death and dying.* New York: Macmillan.

Lakein, A. (1989). *How to get control of your time and your life.* New York: New American Library.

Lerman, L. (1981). *Teaching modern dance to senior citizens: A manual.* Washington, DC: George Washington University.

Lerman, L. (1984). *Teaching dance to senior adults.* Springfield, IL: Charles C Thomas.

Lerner, H.G. (1989). *The dance of anger.* New York: Harper & Row.

Lerner, H.G. (1990). *The dance of intimacy: A woman's guide to courageous acts of change in key relationships.* New York: Harper & Row.

Leslie, D.K. (Ed.). (1990). *Mature stuff: Activities for the older adult.* Reston, VA: American Alliance for Health, Physical Education, Recreation & Dance.

Levine, S. (1982). *Who dies? An investigation of conscious living and dying.* New York: Anchor Books.

Levy, F. (1992). *Dance/movement therapy: A healing art.* Reston, VA: American Alliance for Health, Physical Education, Recreation & Dance.

Lloyd, M. (1990). *Adventures in creative movement activities: A guide to teaching.* Reston, VA: American Alliance for Health, Physical Education, Recreation & Dance.

Lowen, A. (1975). *Bioenergetics.* New York: Penguin Books.

Maas, H.S., & Kuypers, J.A. (1974). *From 30 to 70: A forty-year longitudinal study of adult life styles and personalities.* San Francisco: Jossey-Bass.

MacLennan, B.W., Saul, S., & Weiner, M.B. (Eds.). (1988). *Group psychotherapies for the elderly.* Madison, CT: International Universities Press.

Maiorana, W. (1989). When art is all there is: Art therapy in the treatment of an 80 year old man with Parkinson's disease. *American Journal of Art Therapy, 28*(2), 51–56.

Martz, S.K. (Ed.). (1991). *When I am an old woman I shall wear purple* (2nd ed.). Watsonville, CA: Papier-Mache Press.

McMurray, J. (1989). Creative arts with older people. *Activities, Adaptation and Aging, 14(1/2),* 1–138.

Miller, S., Wackman, D., Nunnally, E., & Saline, C. (1982). *Straight talk: A new way to get close to others by saying what you really mean.* New York: New American Library.

Moen, L. (1992). *Guided imagery* (Vol. II). Naples, FL: United States Publishing.

Montagu, A. (1971). *Touching: The human significance of the skin.* New York: Harper & Row.

Moody, A., Jr. (1978). *Laugh after laugh: The healing power of humor.* Clearwater, FL: Headwaters Press.

Nissenboim, S., & Vroman, C. (1988). *Interactions by design: The positive interactions program for persons with Alzheimer's disease and related disorders.* Crestwood, MO: Geri-Active Consultants.

Oates, W.E. (1985). *Managing your stress.* Philadelphia: Augsburg Fortress.

Oncken, W., Jr. (1986). *Managing management time: Who's got the monkey?* Englewood Cliffs, NJ: Prentice-Hall.

Osgood, N.J., Meyers, B.S., & Orchowsky, S. (1990). The impact of creative dance and movement training on the life satisfaction of older adults: An exploratory study. *Journal of Applied Gerontology, 9,* 255–265.

Ostrow, A.C. (1984). *Physical activity and the older adult.* Reston, VA: American Alliance for Health, Physical Education, Recreation & Dance.

Painter, C. (1985). *Gifts of age: Portraits and essays of 32 remarkable women.* San Francisco: Chronicle Books.

Palmer, M.D. (1977). Music therapy in a comprehensive program of treatment and rehabilitation for the geriatric resident. *Journal of Music Therapy, 14,* 190–197.

Penner, D. (1990). *Elder fit: A health and fitness guide for older adults.* Reston, VA: American Alliance for Health, Physical Education, Recreation & Dance.

Peter, L.J. (1988). *The laughter prescription.* New York: Ballantine Books.

Reader's Digest Editors. (1981). *Family songbook.* Pleasantville, NY: Reader's Digest Association, Inc.

Reader's Digest Editors. (1981). *Treasury of best-loved songs.* Pleasantville, NY: Reader's Digest Association, Inc.

Reader's Digest Editors. (1982). *Popular songs that will live forever.* Pleasantville, NY: Reader's Digest Association, Inc.

Reader's Digest Editors. (1983). *The Reader's Digest country and western songbook.* Pleasantville, NY: Reader's Digest Association, Inc.

Reader's Digest Editors. (1984). *Unforgettable music memories.* Pleasantville, NY: Reader's Digest Association, Inc.

Robey, H. (1982). *There's a dance in the old dame yet.* Boston: Little, Brown.

Robinson, M. (1990). *Humor and the health professions: The therapeutic use of humor in health care* (2nd ed.). Thorofare, NJ: SLACK, Inc.

Roman, S. (1986). *Living with joy: Keys to personal power and spiritual transformation.* Tiburon, CA: H.J. Kramer, Inc.

Ross, R. (1982). *Prospering woman: A complete guide to achieving the full, abundant life.* San Rafael, CA: New World Library.

Schulberg, C. (1981). *The music therapy sourcebook: A collection of activities categorized and analyzed.* New York: Human Sciences Press.

Schweinsberg, M. (1981). Rhythm bands in the nursing home. *Activities, Adaptation and Aging, 1,* 37–41.

Scott, D. (1984). *How to put more time in your life.* New York: New American Library.

Selye, H. (1975). *Stress without distress.* New York: New American Library.

Sher, B., & Gottlieb, A. (1986). *Wishcraft: How to get what you really want.* New York: Ballantine Books.

Sheridan, C. (1987). *Failure-free activities for the Alzheimer's patient: A guide for caregivers.* San Francisco: Elder Books.

Shorr, J. (1977). *Go see the movie in your head.* Santa Barbara, CA: Ross-Erikson.

Siegal, B. (1986). *Love, medicine, and miracles.* New York: Harper & Row.

Simonton, O., Matthews-Simonton, S.M., & Creighton, J. (1978). *Getting well again: A step-by-step self-help guide to overcoming cancer for patients and their families.* New York: J.P. Tarcher.

Stillman, N. (1971). *Trust me with your heart again: A fireside treasury of turn-of-the-century sheet music collected by Norton Stillman.* New York: Simon & Schuster.

Switkes, B. (1982). *Senior-cize: Exercises and dances in a chair.* Silver Spring, MD: Manor Healthcare Corporation.

Tanner, D. (1990). *You just don't understand: Women and men in conversation.* New York: William Morrow.

Tubesing, D.A. (1981). *Kicking your stress habits: A do-it-yourself guide for coping with stress.* Duluth, MN: Whole Person Assocs., Inc.

Van Hugten, C., & De Hullu, O. (1988). *Wheelchair dancing: Rehabilitation, music and human well-being.* St. Louis, MO: MMB Music, Inc.

Van Zandt, S., & Lorenzen, L. (1985). *You're not too old to dance: Creative movement and older adults.* New York: The Haworth Press, Inc.

Walker, S.C. (1994). *Keeping active: A caregiver's guide to activities with the elderly.* Lakewood, CO: American Source Books.

Warren, B. (Ed.). (1984). *Using the creative arts in therapy: A practical introduction.* Cambridge, MA: Brookline Books.

Weinstein, M., & Goodman, J. (1980). *Playfair: Everybody's guide to non-competitive play.* San Luis Obispo, CA: Impact Publishers.

Weissman, J.A. (1983). Planning music activities to meet needs and treatment goals of aged individuals in long-term care facilities. *Music Therapy, 3,* 63–70.

Whitcomb, J.B. (1989). Thanks for the memory. *American Journal of Alzheimer's Care and Related Disorders and Research, 4,* 22–33.

Zgola, J.M. (1987). *Doing things: A guide to programming activities for persons with Alzheimer's disease and related disorders.* Baltimore: Johns Hopkins University Press.

Index

Page numbers followed by "f" indicate figures; numbers followed by "t" indicate tables.